healing foods

healing
foods →

p

This is a Parragon Publishing Book

First published in 2004

Parragon Publishing

Queen Street House

4 Queen Street

Bath BA1 1HE, UK

Produced by The Bridgewater Book Company Ltd

Main photography by Ian Parsons
Home economist: Richard Green

ISBN: 1- 40542-739-6

Printed in Dubai

Wine 1 unit: 8 grams
10 mililiters

contents

→introduction

→ This book concentrates on the latest research, yet the theory that natural foods have therapeutic benefits is hardly new. In the distant past, there was probably little distinction between food and medicine. Today, scientific research into the effects of certain foods on health has supported long-held beliefs that eating the right foods in the right balance can have a positive impact on our health.

→ The foods that are believed to offer specific health benefits have become known as "healing" foods. However, it is important to understand that just because, for example, apples are good for us, it is not beneficial to eat them in excessive quantities. Healing foods should become part of a daily diet that is intrinsically balanced, and which also gives us pleasure.

→ In the chapters that follow, you will find up-to-date information and recipes demonstrating how we can all improve our health and wellbeing. Getting a balance of nutrients is fundamental, and selecting the best ingredients and preparing them in particular ways will ensure that you get the most from your food. In the Looking and Feeling Great sections, we identify which foods make us look and feel good, tackling areas such as skin, hair, and nails, and diseases like heart disease and cancer. The A–Z of Nutritional Healing covers conditions from acne to PMS, explaining how they can be relieved through diet. Finally, the practical Healing Foods Directory enables you to select those foods that will work best for you personally, helping you achieve good health, vitality, and peace of mind.

Fruits and vegetables are nutrient-dense foods, which means that they have a high amount of vitamins and minerals in comparison to the calories they contain. They are generally low in fat, rich in antioxidants, and protect us from the most prevalent diseases.

Try to eat at least 5 portions of fruits and vegetables a day—a mix of different types and colors is preferable.

Balance and variety are the key to planning an optimum diet. This means eating a good range of carbohydrate and protein foods, plenty of fruits and vegetables, and moderate amounts of fat to ensure that you get the nutrients vital for good health.

optimum diet

FRUITS & VEGETABLES

Aim for a minimum of 5 portions a day. A portion equals one medium-sized apple; a banana; 2 plums; a handful of tomatoes; a large bowl of salad; a 3½ oz/100 g slice of melon, 1 cup of raw leafy vegetables, or ½ cup of other vegetables, cooked or chopped raw.

Fruits and vegetables are referred to by nutritionists as "nutrient-dense" foods. This means that they have a high amount of vitamins and minerals in comparison to the calories they contain. They are generally low in fat, rich in antioxidants, known to protect us from the most prevalent diseases, and a good source of fiber. Organic produce—which is grown without the use of chemical fertilizers and pesticides—is becoming increasingly popular and available from stores and markets.

Try to eat a variety of fresh produce in a range of colors, from red and yellow bell peppers, oranges, carrots, and berries to green leafy vegetables such as broccoli, cabbage, cauliflower, and chard, to provide your body with a powerful combination of phytochemicals (see below) and the antioxidants beta carotene and vitamin C.

When cooking vegetables, steaming or stir-frying will retain more nutrients than boiling. Try to eat raw vegetables or salad at least once a day. Freshly squeezed juices have more nutrients than concentrated or long-life alternatives; ¾ cup will account for one of your 5 daily portions. Frozen fruits and vegetables can be just as high in vitamins as fresh, perhaps more so, if the fresh alternative has been stored for some time. Canned produce contains fewer nutrients, and you should opt for no sugar or salt varieties whenever possible.

PHYTOCHEMICALS

RECENT RESEARCH HAS IDENTIFIED A NUMBER OF NATURAL PLANT COMPOUNDS THAT COULD PLAY A CRUCIAL ROLE IN PREVENTING HEART DISEASE, ARTHRITIS, DIABETES, AND CANCER. THESE COMPOUNDS ARE KNOWN COLLECTIVELY AS PHYTOCHEMICALS AND MAY, IN THE FUTURE, BE CLASSIFIED AS ESSENTIAL NUTRIENTS. FRUITS AND VEGETABLES, WHOLE GRAINS, NUTS, SEEDS, DRIED BEANS, AND LENTILS CONTAIN A RANGE OF PHYTOCHEMICALS.

Around 50 percent of our daily diet should be made up of carbohydrate foods and they should form a part of every meal, since they supply the body with the sustained energy that it needs to function effectively.

All carbohydrate foods provide sustained energy. Unrefined varieties are richer in nutrients and fiber.

WHOLE GRAINS, CEREALS, AND POTATOES

Aim for 6–11 servings a day. A portion is a slice of bread, a bowl of cereal, 1 medium potato, or ½ cup cooked cereal, rice, or pasta.

This group includes cereals, bread, rice, noodles, pasta, and potatoes, otherwise known as carbohydrate or starchy foods. Some 50 percent of our daily diet should be made up of these foods. They should form a part of every meal, since they supply the body with the sustained energy that it needs to function effectively.

The more unrefined the better. Foods containing refined and processed grains and cereals not only contain fewer nutrients but lead to yo-yoing blood sugar levels, the effects of which are mood swings and variation in energy levels. Whole-wheat is better than white, because these foods provide more fiber, B-group vitamins, and minerals (see Vitamin and Mineral table on pages 20–23). Fiber helps to protect against digestive disorders and heart disease and comes in two forms: insoluble fiber helps to prevent constipation and bowel disorders by speeding up the passage of food through the large intestine. Whole wheat, brown rice, and nuts are good sources of insoluble fiber. Soluble fiber, found mainly in beans, vegetables, and oats, can reduce harmful blood cholesterol and help control blood sugar levels.

Carbohydrate foods are often accused of being fattening but it tends to be what you serve with them, such as butter, cheese, or creamy sauces, that bumps up the calories and fat levels.

Protein is vital for growth and repair. Eat moderate amounts daily to ensure you get a complete range of essential amino acids.

MEAT, FISH, AND PROTEIN ALTERNATIVES

Aim for 2–3 servings a day. A serving equals 2–3 oz/ 55–75 g cooked lean meat, poultry, or fish; 2 eggs; 1 cup cooked dried beans, or 2 tbsp nuts.

Moderate amounts of lean meat, poultry, fish, Quorn™, eggs, dried beans and lentils, nuts, seeds, and tofu are recommended on a daily basis, but try to eat a variety to ensure a good balance of amino acids. This group of foods is essential for growth, repair, and maintenance in the body, and provides valuable amounts of iron, B-group vitamins, zinc, magnesium, vitamin E, and fiber.

The body requires protein in relatively small amounts, so foods from this group should make up around only 10–12 percent of the daily diet. Limit red meat to 3 servings a week and try to eat oily fish, such as

sardines, tuna, salmon, herring, and mackerel, twice a week. These fish contain rich amounts of omega-3 fatty acids, which are thought to reduce the risk of heart disease. Limit your egg intake to 4 a week.

Since animal sources of protein can be high in fat, it is important to balance this with plant forms found in beans, peas, and lentils. These are low in fat and high in fiber. Nuts and seeds are nutritious, a good source of the essential fatty acid omega-6, yet are relatively high in fat, so eat on a regular basis but in moderate amounts.

The high-protein diets that are currently fashionable may not be good for you in the long term. Studies have found a link between a high-protein diet and constipation, bowel disease, and an increased risk of osteoporosis, since in excess protein encourages the excretion of calcium from the bones. Also, too much protein in the long term may affect kidney function.

Eat a good range of carbohydrate and protein foods,

plenty of fruits and vegetables, and moderate amounts

of fat to ensure that you get the nutrients vital for health.

*Low-fat dairy foods
and fats are the
healthiest option.*

recommended that children under the age of two should not be given low-fat dairy produce such as lowfat milk. Children over two years can be given lowfat milk but not skim milk, providing they are eating a varied, balanced diet.

Organic dairy produce is preferable as it is free from antibiotic residues, growth hormones, and agrochemicals. Soy, oat, or rice milk make good alternatives to cow's milk and are also a good source of calcium.

MILK & DAIRY FOODS

Aim for 2–3 servings a day. A serving equals 1 cup of milk or yogurt or 1½ oz/40 g natural cheese, such as Cheddar.

Milk, cheese, and yogurt provide valuable amounts of protein, calcium, some B-group vitamins, including B_{12}, B_6, and B_2, as well as vitamins A and D, essential for healthy teeth and bones and the release of energy from food. Nutritionists advise that this group of foods should make up about 15 percent of our daily diet.

Dairy produce, particularly hard cheese, can be high in saturated fat, so opt for low-fat varieties. Children, however, need a certain amount of fat, and it is

FATS

Aim to eat sparingly.

A certain amount of fat is necessary for good health—in fact, too little has been linked to depression—but it is essential to eat the right type. Fat is mainly used by the body as energy, providing and transporting vitamins A, D, E, and K around the body. Official dietary guidelines recommend that fats should make up no more than 30 percent of total calories.

There are two main types of fat: saturated and unsaturated. There is a proven link between too much saturated fat and high cholesterol, plus an increased risk of heart disease, cancer, and obesity. It is important to minimize intake of animal fats in particular, including meat, cheese, cream, and butter, and opt for lean and

*Choose live plain bio yogurt
to help maintain a healthy
intestinal environment.*

low-fat versions. Saturated fat is also found in milk chocolate, cookies, and cakes. Margarine, once hailed as the healthy alternative to butter, is often laden with additives, preservatives, and hydrogenated or trans fats, which have been found to be even worse for your health than saturated fat. When buying margarine, look for those that are non-hydrogenated. This type of fat is also often found in processed foods.

Unsaturated fats, both polyunsaturated and monounsaturated, can help to reduce harmful "LDL" (Low Density Lipoprotein) cholesterol—the type that furs up the arteries. Polyunsaturated fats provide the essential fatty acids, omega-3 and omega-6. Oily fish, walnuts, soybeans, and rape seeds provide omega-3, while omega-6 is found in vegetable oils, nuts, and seeds.

Essential fatty acids have been found to reduce the risk of heart disease, cancer, skin complaints, arthritis, and PMS. Monounsaturated fat, found in olive oil, canola oil, olives, and avocados, not only reduces harmful LDL cholesterol in the body but maintains or raises good "HDL" (High Density Lipoprotein) cholesterol levels. There is also a link between mono-unsaturated fat and a reduced risk of heart disease and cancer, along with increased life expectancy.

Oily fish contain essential fatty acids, which reduce your risk of heart disease and cancer.

Try to drink 6–8 glasses (1½–1¾ quarts) of water a day.

WATER

Water plays a vital role in maintaining good health but few of us drink enough. It delivers nutrients around the body, regulates body temperature, and transports waste. It is best to choose filtered or natural mineral water to achieve the desired daily amount. Coffee, tea, and soda contain caffeine, which has a diuretic effect, so they actually dehydrate the body. Herbal or rooibosch (red) tea are healthy, caffeine-free alternatives.

The way you buy, store, and prepare your food can affect its nutritional status. The following tips will help you get the most from your food.

BUYING TIPS

⊙ Whenever possible, buy organic, seasonal, and local produce. You may have to pay slightly more, but the foods are usually fresher, more nutritious, and less damaging to the environment than foods flown thousands of miles and kept in cold storage for months.

optimize your foods

⊙ Buying from a local market or producer, or direct from a farm is a good way to source fresh produce—it can also be cheaper.

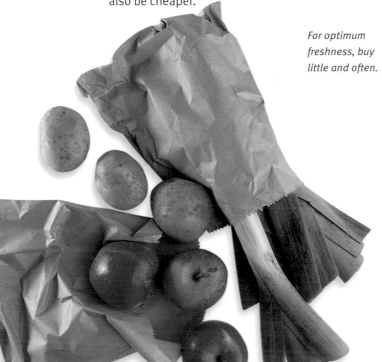

For optimum freshness, buy little and often.

⊙ Buy fresh foods from stores with a high turnover of goods. Avoid fruits and vegetables that are displayed in the open air or in a hot, light window, since nutrients will be diminished. Fluorescent lighting also depletes nutrients.

⊙ Buy fresh produce in small quantities on a regular basis and remove them from plastic bags when storing. Loose fresh produce is also much easier to check for quality.

⊙ Purchase or choose chilled and frozen foods last to keep them cool and to avoid spoilage and possible growth of bacteria.

⊙ When buying fresh meat, fish, and shellfish, it is easier to check quality and freshness if buying over the counter. Wild or organic salmon and trout are preferable to farmed fish. Undyed smoked haddock and cod is better than the highly colored, bright yellow alternatives.

⊙ Check labels when buying packaged foods. Avoid those with high amounts of sugar, saturated and hydrogenated (trans) fat, colors, additives, flavoring, preservatives, and artificial sweeteners.

⊙ When buying eggs, look for organic, high-quality ones. Farm-fresh or boxes depicting attractive countryside scenes mean nothing: the eggs are usually from battery farms. Organic eggs come from hens that have been better looked after, and are not routinely fed antibiotics or yolk-enhancing dyes.

Whenever possible, buy local produce in season.

● The terms "natural", "country", or "traditional" mean little when used on processed foods.

● You pay for what you get—if buying processed foods, opt for good quality such as burgers and sausages with a high meat content and minimum amount of fat and fillers. Choose fish or poultry without crumb or other coatings, which can be an excuse for manufacturers to add colors, preservatives, fat, and cheap fillers.

● Check labels for Food Safety and Inspection Services/FDA approval of production standards and quality of ingredients, when buying meat and poultry.

STORING & COOKING TIPS

● Depending on the type of fruit or vegetable, store in a cool pantry or in the bottom of the refrigerator. Avoid keeping them for too long, since nutrients diminish with age. Some fruits such as bananas, melons, peaches, and avocados can be ripened at room temperature.

● Raw fruits and vegetables are generally the most nutritious. Avoid peeling them, if possible, since many nutrients are found in or just below the skin.

● Do not prepare fruits and vegetables too far in advance of cooking or serving as nutrients diminish as soon as cut surfaces are exposed to the air.

● Steaming is preferable to boiling—the latter destroys water-soluble vitamins such as C and B-complex. Stir-frying is another good way of retaining nutrients. If you boil vegetables, use as little water as possible and do not overcook them. The cooking water can also be kept and used to make stock for soup or sauces.

● Buy nuts and seeds in small quantities and store in an airtight container in a cool, dark cupboard. Don't keep them for too long as they can become rancid. Herbs, spices, dried beans and lentils, flour, and grains should be kept in the same way.

● Store oils in a cool, dark place to prevent oxidation.

optimize your foods

Deciding which foods to cut back on is just as crucial as what you choose to include in your diet. Foods high in sugar, fat, and salt provide the body with negligible nutrients and can do more harm than good.

SUGAR

Refined sugars and those found in processed foods, including cookies, candy, and cakes, have little or no nutritional value. Eating a sugary food gives a temporary surge in energy, which is promptly followed by a slump.

what to avoid

It is this fluctuation in blood sugar levels that leads to an inconsistent supply of energy to the brain, leading to poor concentration, mood swings, brain "fug", and tiredness. Many sweet foods combine sugar with fat, so tooth decay and weight gain are both consequences of eating too much of these foods.

Moderation is the key. Don't deny yourself completely, but try to restrict eating sweet foods to after a meal to avoid swings in blood sugar. Look out for sucrose, fructose, glucose, maltose, corn syrup, invert sugar, and dextrose on food labels, which are basically sugar by another name. Honey and maple syrup are marginally better as they contain a few minerals, but they have the same effect on blood sugar levels.

Recent studies show that sugar has an aging effect on the skin—not to mention the detrimental effect on teeth and weight.

A bowl of cornflakes contains more salt than a packet of potato chips.

Many low-sugar foods contain artificial sweeteners, such as saccharin or aspartame, which have been linked to hyperactivity in children as well as diarrhea if eaten in excess. They also perpetuate a sweet tooth.

SALT

On average, Americans eat 10 g of salt a day—5 g is the upper recommended amount—most of which is found in processed foods. Potato chips, crackers, salted nuts, bouillon cubes, packaged soups, and cheese are obvious culprits but, surprisingly, a bowl of cornflakes is higher in salt than a bag of potato chips. Other processed foods that contain high amounts of salt include cookies, baked beans, and bread. The salt we need is supplied in adequate amounts in natural foods such as meat, fish, and vegetables. Excess salt is a major cause of high blood pressure, which leads to strokes and heart attacks. Too much salt in the diet has also been linked to fluid retention and kidney stones.

CAFFEINE

Caffeine is a stimulant, which means it helps to keep us alert and awake. If drunk in excess (over 8 cups a day), however, it can lead to the jitters, shakes, headaches, an irregular heartbeat, and stomach upsets. It is also a diuretic, causing dehydration in the body. Those at risk of osteoporosis should pay special attention to their caffeine intake, since it increases the excretion of

Herb teas are naturally caffeine-free.

calcium in the urine. It also inhibits the absorption of vitamins and minerals from the gut.

Coffee contains about 40 percent more caffeine than tea and chocolate. Strong Continental European brands are more likely to have noticeable side effects. Soda, such as cola, also contains caffeine. Try to limit yourself to no more than three caffeine drinks a day. Herbal teas and coffee alternatives are healthier options.

Moderation is the key. Try to restrict eating sweet foods

to after a meal, reduce your salt and caffeine intake, and

limit your alcohol intake to 14 units a week for women

and 21 units a week for men.

Heavy drinking can lead to depression, insomnia, anxiety, and forgetfulness. It can also increase the risk of osteoporosis, certain cancers, heart disease, impotence, and brain and liver damage in the long term. Alcohol is an appetite suppressant, so those who drink too much risk being deficient in nutrients. Additionally, alcohol affects the absorption of vitamins A, B, C, and D, essential fatty acids, calcium, zinc, magnesium, and phosphorus.

If drunk in excess, alcohol affects the absorption of nutrients from food.

ALCOHOL

The latest research shows that not all alcohol is bad for you. Red wine, for example, has been found to help prevent heart attacks. Antioxidants known as flavonols are the key, since they help to make the blood less prone to clotting. Antioxidants also help to mop up harmful free radicals in the body by reducing cell damage, known to cause cancer. Whiskey is also said to raise antioxidant levels.

Moderation, however, is vital. Although drinking around two units of wine or beer a day may reduce the risk of heart disease, women should not exceed 14 units of alcohol a week, men 21 units. Avoid binge drinking and spread your intake throughout the week, keeping two consecutive days completely alcohol-free.

The long-term effects of pesticide use are unknown.

ADDITIVES

The most commonly used additives are colors, preservatives, flavor enhancers, emulsifiers, flavorings, and glazing agents. Not all additives are potentially harmful, but some have been linked to hyperactivity in children, poor memory, depression, and mood swings.

Although additives have to be listed on food labels, it is not easy to avoid them altogether. The flavor enhancer monosodium glutamate (commonly known as MSG), for example, is routinely added to flavored potato chips. MSG has been linked to a range of symptoms, including dizziness, anxiety, mood swings, pain in the chest, palpitations, sweating, headaches, and asthma attacks. The simplest option is to reduce the amount of processed foods you buy, opting for fresh, unadulterated foods instead.

buying good-quality, fresh produce that does not look old, wilted, or moldy. Wash all fruits and vegetables thoroughly, including prewashed salads, before cooking or serving raw. Remove the outer leaves of vegetables or trim and peel them. Scrub the skin of hard fruits such as melon before preparing them. By following these guidelines, you should succeed in removing half to three-quarters of whatever residue remains on your fruits and vegetables.

PESTICIDES

Despite government reassurances that pesticides used in agriculture do not exceed legal limits, we do not know enough about the long-term effects of ingesting small doses of pesticides, nor the possible danger to the body of eating these different pesticides in combination.

Common pesticides include organophosphates, herbicides, fungicides, nitrates, and growth regulators. Buying organic produce is one way to help avoid them. You can also reduce your chances of residue intake by

Wash all fruits and vegetables thoroughly before use.

Fruits and vegetables are obvious sources of nutrients, but a diet incorporating all food types is essential to gain a good balance of vitamins and minerals.

essential vitamins & minerals

A varied and balanced diet is the key to good health.

VITAMIN

A (retinol in animal foods, beta carotene in plant foods)

B1 (thiamine)

B2 (riboflavin)

B3 (niacin)

B6 (pyridoxine)

B12 (cyanocobalamin)

Folate (folic acid)

C (ascorbic acid)

⊕ **BEST SOURCES**	⊕ **ROLE IN HEALTH**	⊗ **DEFICIENCY**
➲ Animal sources: milk, butter, cheese, egg yolk, margarine, and liver. Plant sources: carrots, apricots, squash, red bell peppers, broccoli, green leafy vegetables, mango, and sweet potatoes	⊕ Necessary for vision, bone growth, skin, and tissue repair. Beta carotene acts as an antioxidant and protects the immune system	⊗ Poor night vision, dry skin, and lower resistance to infection, especially respiratory disorders
➲ Whole-grain cereals, brewer's yeast, potatoes, yeast extract, nuts, dried beans and lentils, and Quorn™	⊕ Essential for energy production, the nervous system, muscles, and the heart; promotes growth and boosts mental wellbeing	⊗ Depression, irritability, nervous disorders, loss of memory. Common among alcoholics
➲ Cheese, eggs, milk, yogurt, fortified breakfast cereals, yeast extract, almonds, and pumpkin seeds	⊕ Vital for energy production, tissue repair, and maintenance, and the functioning of vitamin B_6 and niacin	⊗ Lack of energy, dry cracked lips, numbness, and itchy eyes
➲ Dried beans and lentils, potatoes, fortified breakfast cereals, wheat germ, peanuts, cheese, eggs, mushrooms, green leafy vegetables, figs, prunes, poultry, tuna, and pork	⊕ Essential for a healthy digestive system, skin, and circulation. Also needed to release energy from food	⊗ Deficiency is unusual but is characterized by lack of energy, depression, and scaly skin
➲ Eggs, wheat germ, whole-wheat bread, breakfast cereals, nuts, bananas, poultry, salmon, and lentils	⊕ Assimilates protein and fat to make red blood cells; maintains a healthy immune system	⊗ Anemia, dermatitis, and depression
➲ Milk, eggs, fortified breakfast cereals, cheese, yeast extract, liver, mussels, oily fish, and lean beef	⊕ Required in the formation of red blood cells, maintaining a healthy nervous system, and energy production	⊗ Fatigue, increased risk of infection, anemia
➲ Green leafy vegetables, fortified breakfast cereals, bread, nuts, dried beans and lentils, bananas, yeast extract, and asparagus	⊕ Vital for cell division (growth). An increased intake is recommended pre-conception and during the first three months of pregnancy to protect the fetus against neural tube defects	⊗ Anemia and appetite loss. Linked to neural defects in babies
➲ Citrus fruits, melons, strawberries, tomatoes, broccoli, potatoes, bell peppers, and green vegetables	⊕ Helps the body absorb iron, and maintains healthy skin, teeth, and bones. An antioxidant that strengthens the immune system and helps fight infection	⊗ Increased susceptibility to infection, fatigue, poor sleep, and depression

essential vitamins & minerals

Keeping active is as important as a good diet for maintaining health.

Many nutrients in fruits and vegetables are found in or just below the skin, so prepare them carefully to maximize nutrition.

Fresh, unprocessed foods provide a range of beneficial, therapeutic nutrients.

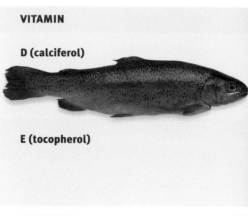

VITAMIN

D (calciferol)

E (tocopherol)

MINERAL

Calcium

Iron

Zinc

Potassium

Magnesium

Phosphorus

Selenium

→ Margarine, vegetable oils, eggs, cereals, butter, cod liver oil, and oily fish. Also sunlight

→ Seeds, wheat germ, nuts, vegetable oils, eggs, whole-wheat bread, green leafy vegetables, oats, sunflower oil, avocados, and fortified breakfast cereals

⊕ **ROLE IN HEALTH**

⊕ Helps the body to absorb calcium and phosphorus, which is vital for bone and teeth formation

⊕ An antioxidant that is essential for healthy skin, circulation, and maintaining cells

⊗ **DEFICIENCY**

⊗ Softening of the bones and muscle weakness. Long-term shortage results in rickets

⊗ Increased risk of heart attack, stroke, and some cancers

→ **BEST SOURCES**

→ Milk, cheese, yogurt, green leafy vegetables, sesame seeds, broccoli, dried figs, dried beans and lentils, almonds, spinach, watercress, sardines, and tofu

→ Egg yolk, fortified breakfast cereals, green leafy vegetables, dried apricots, prunes, dried beans and lentils, whole grains, tofu, seeds, beef, liver, brown rice

→ Peanuts, whole grains, sunflower and pumpkin seeds, dried beans, lentils, milk, hard cheese, yogurt, wheat germ, liver, Quorn™, crab, lamb, beef

→ Bananas, milk, dried beans and lentils, nuts, seeds, whole grains, potatoes, fruits, and vegetables

→ Nuts, seeds, whole grains, dried beans and lentils, tofu, dried figs, dried apricots, and green vegetables

→ Milk, cheese, yogurt, eggs, nuts, seeds, dried beans and lentils, whole grains, meat, and fish

→ Avocados, lentils, milk, cheese, butter, brazil nuts, seaweed, tuna, white fish, sardines, salmon, and pork

⊕ **ROLE IN HEALTH**

⊕ Builds and maintains bones and teeth; maintains muscle function and the nervous system

⊕ Carries oxygen from the lungs to all the cells in the body

⊕ Essential for a healthy immune system, tissue formation, normal growth, wound healing, and reproduction

⊕ Regulates body fluids and maintains normal blood pressure and nerve transmission

⊕ Keeps muscles, bones, and teeth healthy. Required for normal growth and nerve formation

⊕ Essential for healthy bones and teeth, energy production, and the assimilation of nutrients, particularly calcium

⊕ An antioxidant that protects against cancer, heart disease, and premature aging

⊗ **DEFICIENCY**

⊗ Soft and brittle bones, osteoporosis, fractures, and muscle weakness

⊗ Anemia, fatigue, and low resistance to infection

⊗ Impaired growth and development, slow wound healing, and loss of taste and smell

⊗ Weakness, thirst, fatigue, mental confusion, and raised blood pressure

⊗ Lethargy, weak bones and muscles, depression, and irritability

⊗ Deficiency is rare

⊗ Reduced antioxidant protection

essential vitamins & minerals

→looking great

A healthy outer self is an excellent indication of inner health, and knowing that you look great is a wonderful confidence booster. This chapter looks at the foods that can improve the condition of skin, hair, teeth, and nails, alongside useful recipes and advice on complementary remedies.

The skin is one of the major organs responsible for eliminating toxic waste. The single most important nutrient, vital for hydrating the skin and flushing out toxins, is water.

skin

We all want a glowing, healthy, blemish-free complexion. When your skin looks good, you feel good—an excellent reason to give it a boost through a well-balanced diet.

Stress, environmental pollution, sun, and lack of sleep all take their toll on our skin and, of course, genetic make-up plays a part. Poor digestion, food intolerances, and allergies can also cause or exacerbate skin disorders, such as acne, eczema, and psoriasis. But eating the right foods and drinking plenty of water can improve and revitalize the skin, helping to relieve existing skin problems and curbing the onset of others. The skin is one of the major organs responsible for eliminating waste. A diet high in junk foods, laced with alcohol and cigarettes, means that it has to work harder to get rid of toxic waste products and can be overloaded with harmful toxins.

The single most important nutrient for a glowing complexion is water. We should drink about 6–8 glasses a day to hydrate the skin and help flush out toxins. Other essential nutrients include vitamin A, which combats dryness and keeps skin soft; B-group vitamins to promote a glowing complexion and aid the renewal of skin cells; vitamin C to strengthen blood vessels and maintain collagen and elastin levels; vitamin E to transport nutrients to the skin cells and reduce damage by harmful free radicals; zinc to improve skin tone, encourage healing, and prevent skin infections; and essential fatty acids, which contain high levels of the skin-tightening chemical dimethylaminoethanol (DMAE), so helping to maintain collagen and elastin levels, hydrate, firm, and boost skin tone.

SKIN TIPS

➕ SPEND 5 MINUTES A DAY BRUSHING YOUR BODY IN LONG, SWEEPING MOTIONS, ALWAYS TOWARD THE HEART. SKIN BRUSHING IMPROVES LYMPHATIC DRAINAGE AND SLUGGISH CIRCULATION, SHIFTING STUBBORN CELLULITE.

USEFUL FOODS

✅ Carrots, broccoli, spinach, sweet potatoes, pumpkin, and apricots are all rich in beta carotene, which counters dry, flaky skin.

✅ Apples, artichokes, beets, and asparagus cleanse the liver and kidneys, helping to detoxify the skin.

✅ Avocados provide vitamins A, C, and E, and valuable monounsaturated fat, which helps to keep the skin supple.

✅ Essential fatty acids found in oily fish and linseeds (omega-3), as well as nuts and seeds (omega-6), soften and hydrate the skin and protect against sun damage.

AVOID

❌ Alcohol dehydrates the skin, creates harmful free radicals, and depletes the skin of certain vitamins, particularly B-group and C. Additionally, it weakens blood capillaries, leading to thread veins.

❌ Smoking depletes vitamin C, causing the blood vessels to constrict and slowing down circulation.

❌ Processed foods provide few nutrients and are often loaded with chemical additives, colors, and preservatives.

❌ Saturated and hydrogenated fats slow down the lymphatic system, essential for the transport of nutrients, and generate high levels of destructive free radicals.

❌ Refined sugar, believed to be as harmful as tobacco, affects skin elasticity, leading to wrinkles and skin aging.

guacamole with roasted vegetables

This creamy dip is an excellent source of the antioxidants, vitamins C and E, and avocado has the highest protein content of any fruit.

Serves 2

Ingredients
1 avocado, pitted
1 small garlic clove, crushed
1 tbsp fresh lemon juice

Roasted vegetables
**Choose from a selection of butternut
 squash, red bell pepper, asparagus,
 red onion, zucchini, carrots, and
 fennel, cut into chunks**
1 tbsp olive oil
few sprigs fresh rosemary

❶

Preheat the oven to 400°F/200°C. Place your chosen selection of vegetables in a roasting dish. Toss the vegetables in the olive oil using your hands. Place the sprigs of rosemary on top and roast in the oven for 30–40 minutes until the vegetables are tender and golden.

❷

Meanwhile, make the guacamole. Scoop out the avocado flesh using a spoon. Mash with the garlic and lemon juice until fairly smooth and creamy.

❸

To serve, remove the rosemary sprigs and arrange the roasted vegetables on a plate. Top with a spoonful of guacamole. Serve with whole-wheat pita bread.

27

Overexposure to hair dyes and perming lotions sometimes causes hair and scalp problems, but a healthy, balanced diet will help to rectify the damage and boost condition.

hair

Dull, lackluster hair may be an indication that you are lacking in nutrients. There is a correlation between the state of your hair and your inner health and general wellbeing. Illness, stress, or an emotional problem can all have a detrimental effect on your hair condition, which even a good haircut and the latest styling products won't be able to remedy. Overexposure to hair dyes and perming lotions sometimes causes hair and scalp problems, but a healthy, balanced diet will help to rectify the damage and boost condition.

The B-group vitamins as well as vitamins C and E, beta carotene, iron, zinc, and selenium help to feed the hair and are of prime importance. Drinking plenty of mineral or filtered water—about 6–8 glasses a day—can also improve the condition of your hair. Stress can have a damaging effect on hair condition, causing scalp disorders such as dandruff. Since people suffering from stress are likely to be short of B-group vitamins, it is particularly important to include sufficient amounts of whole grains, lean meat, poultry, eggs, nuts, and dried beans and lentils in the diet. Zinc is said to alleviate dandruff, and is found in shellfish, dairy products, whole-grain bread, and cereals.

Significant hair loss has been linked to low iron levels. If you need to boost your intake of this mineral, increase your intake of vitamin C at the same time as this will help your body absorb the iron. Biotin deficiency can also contribute to hair loss. Although this nutrient is mainly produced by bacteria in the gut, it is also found in cooked eggs, peanut butter, liver, and whole grains.

USEFUL FOODS

- ✓ In Japan, a diet rich in seaweed is believed to give you lustrous hair, probably on account of its high mineral content.
- ✓ Essential fatty acids found in oily fish, vegetable oils, nuts, and seeds can help prevent a dry, flaky scalp.
- ✓ Lean red meat, eggs, dried beans and lentils, dried apricots, and green leafy vegetables are a good source of iron, which helps counter hair loss.
- ✓ Protein is vital for hair growth, making it shiny and keeping it in good condition. Opt for lean meat, chicken, fish, eggs, low-fat dairy products, dried beans and lentils, nuts, and seeds.

AVOID

- ✗ Caffeine, found in coffee, tea, and some soda, dehydrates the body and inhibits the absorption of certain nutrients, including iron.
- ✗ Smoking reduces vitamin C levels in the body, which is vital for healthy hair.
- ✗ Refined carbohydrates such as white bread, pasta, and rice are robbed of many of their beneficial nutrients during processing. Choose unrefined whole-wheat bread and pasta and brown rice instead.
- ✗ Alternative practitioners recommend cutting down on sugar to prevent oily hair.

Keep your locks shiny and glossy by including protein foods in your diet.

RECIPE

japanese salad

This salad contains arame, a mild-tasting seaweed, which is rich in the minerals necessary for glossy hair. You can buy it at the larger supermarkets, Asian markets, or health food shops.

Serves 2

Ingredients

½ oz/15 g arame

4 oz/115 g radishes, thinly sliced into rounds

½ small cucumber, cut into thin sticks

1 cup bean sprouts, rinsed

sesame seeds, for sprinkling

Dressing

1 tbsp sunflower oil

1 tsp toasted sesame oil

2 tsp white wine vinegar

½ tsp soy sauce

1

Rinse the arame in a strainer under cold running water. Place in a bowl and cover with more cold water. Let soak for 5 minutes—the arame should double in volume. Drain and place in a pan.

2

Cover the arame with cold water and bring to a boil. Reduce the heat and simmer for 20 minutes until tender, then drain.

3

Meanwhile, mix all the ingredients for the dressing together in a bowl.

4

Combine the arame with the radishes, cucumber, and bean sprouts. Spoon over the dressing and sprinkle with sesame seeds before serving.

HAIR TIPS

✚ BREWER'S YEAST, WHICH YOU CAN BUY AT ANY HEALTH FOOD SHOP, IS RECOMMENDED FOR PEOPLE WITH HAIR PROBLEMS. IT IS AN EXCELLENT SOURCE OF B-GROUP VITAMINS, IRON, ZINC, AND OTHER MINERALS.

It is important to instill good habits early to ensure healthy teeth throughout life. Good care and maintenance of baby teeth helps to ensure the development of healthy adult teeth.

teeth

A healthy diet is just as important as regular brushing and good dental hygiene when it comes to having white, clean, strong teeth.

While general dental health is better than it was in the past, we can all improve the condition of our teeth through brushing and flossing every day and eating certain foods. It is important to instill good habits early to ensure healthy teeth throughout life. Although the first set of baby teeth or "milk teeth" are temporary, a range of nutrients and dental care are still necessary to build and maintain them. Their health also affects the development of adult teeth.

Healthy teeth require the same nutrients as strong bones, namely calcium, magnesium, and vitamin D. Looking after your gums is also essential. Foods rich in B-group vitamins, beta carotene, vitamin C, zinc, and folic acid will all help keep them healthy. Mouth ulcers are a sign that the immune system is compromised and that the body may be lacking in essential nutrients.

Sugar is the biggest enemy of teeth, and it is the frequency that it is eaten that increases the likelihood of tooth decay. Sugar is not only present in cakes, candy, cookies, and soda, but is found in many forms and in many types of food, including savory ones. Check labels for the following: fructose, sucrose, dextrose, glucose, syrup, maltose, and concentrated fruit juice. Choose savory foods as snacks, such as vegetables, bread, and cheese. Fruits are also good for teeth. However, since they contain natural sugars and are acidic, you should rinse your mouth with water after eating. Foods that require chewing help to keep teeth and gums healthy.

Calcium is as essential for healthy teeth as it is for strong bones.

USEFUL FOODS

- ✓ Dairy products including cheese, milk, and yogurt are an excellent source of calcium.
- ✓ Apricots, nuts (especially almonds), seeds, tofu, sardines, shrimp, broccoli, and dark-green leafy vegetables are valuable non-dairy sources of calcium.
- ✓ Magnesium, important for strong bones and teeth, is found in whole grains, dried fruits, nuts, seeds, dried beans, lentils, and green leafy vegetables.

AVOID

- ✗ Sugar in all its various forms is the number one cause of tooth decay.
- ✗ Honey is as damaging to your teeth as sugar, although it does have some therapeutic properties.
- ✗ Soda, fruit juices, cordials, and some fruit and herbal teas contain sugar. A glass of fruit juice contains beneficial vitamins, but dilute it with water to reduce its sugar content.
- ✗ Dairy and wheat have been known to trigger food allergies and intolerances, leading to bad breath. Consult your health adviser before eliminating these foods.

raspberry and oat crunch

This pudding looks stunning but is very simple to make. It also makes a nutritious breakfast, providing useful amounts of calcium, and vitamins B and C.

Serves 2

Ingredients

½ cup whole porridge oats

1 tbsp sunflower seeds

1 cup fresh or frozen raspberries (defrost before using)

1¼ cups thick live plain bio yogurt

1 tbsp honey or maple syrup

Place the porridge oats and sunflower seeds in a large, heavy-bottomed skillet and roast over medium heat for 1–2 minutes until lightly toasted. Let cool.

Place the yogurt in a large bowl and stir in the honey or maple syrup. Add the raspberries and fold in gently.

❸
Stir in the oats and sunflower seeds, leaving a few to sprinkle on top. Spoon the mixture into 2 glasses and top with the oats and seeds before serving.

TEETH TIPS

✛ COENZYME Q-10, FOUND IN SARDINES, MACKEREL, PORK, SPINACH, PEANUTS, SOYBEAN OIL, AND SESAME SEEDS, IS ESSENTIAL FOR THE PRODUCTION OF ENERGY AND HELPS COMBAT GUM DISEASE.

looking great

Nails are made of a protein called keratin and should be strong, smooth, and pink. Pale, brittle, or ridged nails are usually a sign of vitamin and/or mineral deficiency.

nails

The health of your skin and hair is reflected in the condition of your nails. Since all benefit from a well-balanced diet, it is important to ensure that you eat a range of different foods.

Nails are made of a protein called keratin and should be strong, smooth, and pink. Pale, brittle, or ridged nails may be a sign of iron or zinc deficiency. If you suspect you are anemic, ask your health adviser for a blood test, and boost your intake of iron-rich foods. Eat plenty of vitamin C-rich foods at the same time to help your body absorb the iron. Lack of selenium, found in fish, shellfish, offal, grains, and cereals, can also lead to ridged nails. White spots on the nails may be an indication of zinc deficiency, although they can also be the result of a knock.

A low-protein diet will adversely affect the condition of your nails. Not only does protein provide essential amino acids, it also encourages the absorption of iron. Meat, poultry, seafood, eggs, dairy products, nuts, dried beans, and lentils contain a good range of essential amino acids. Try to eat a variety in your diet, but opt for low-fat versions where possible. A deficiency of biotin, a nutrient mainly produced by bacteria in the intestine, will also affect your nails. It is found in cooked eggs, whole grains, peanut butter, and liver. A shortage of B-group vitamins may lead to ridged nails—eat whole grains, dairy foods, dried beans, lentils, seafood, meat, nuts, seeds, green vegetables, and yeast extract.

Citrus fruits, such as oranges, provide vitamin C which aids the absorption of iron, vital for strong nails.

USEFUL FOODS

- Citrus fruits, green leafy vegetables, black currants, bell peppers, tomatoes, and potatoes provide useful amounts of vitamin C, which helps the body absorb iron.
- Oysters and other shellfish, seeds, dried beans and lentils, lean meat, and dairy foods are rich in zinc, which helps prevent brittle nails.
- Iron is found in offal, red meat, oily fish, mussels, dried apricots, green leafy vegetables, dried beans and lentils, and tofu.

AVOID

- Tea contains tannin, which inhibits the absorption of iron. Brittle, pale nails may indicate iron deficiency.
- Heavy drinking dehydrates the body, depletes it of vital vitamins, and impairs its ability to absorb protein.
- Smoking affects the body's ability to metabolize vitamin C, essential for strong nails, and inhibits the transport of oxygen and other nutrients throughout the body.

RECIPE

spicy mussels

Zinc, iron, and vitamin C are found in beneficial amounts in this aromatic shellfish dish. Serve with plenty of crusty bread.

Serves 2

Ingredients

1 tbsp olive oil

1 onion, finely chopped

2 garlic cloves, crushed

1 cup dry white wine

4 tbsp canned chopped tomatoes

1 tbsp chopped flatleaf parsley

¼ tsp dried chili flakes

2 lb 4 oz/1 kg mussels, scrubbed, cleaned, and rinsed

squeeze of fresh lemon juice

black pepper

Heat the oil in a large, deep pan. Add the onion and cook for 8 minutes over medium heat until softened. Add the garlic. Cook for an additional minute, stirring frequently.

2

Increase the heat, add the wine, and boil for 2 minutes until reduced. Reduce the heat to medium and add the tomatoes, parsley, and chili flakes. Simmer for 5 minutes or until reduced by a third.

3

Toss in the mussels, cover the pan, and cook for 5 minutes or until the mussels have opened. Shake the pan occasionally. Discard any mussels that remain closed.

4

Add a squeeze of lemon juice and season with black pepper. Spoon into large bowls and serve immediately.

→feeling great

Eating the right foods can reduce your risk of cancer and heart disease as well as improve your memory and increase energy levels. This chapter looks at the foods we should include in our diet and those that are best avoided. There are more recipes to try plus further advice on complementary remedies.

Most experts agree that dietary changes can lessen your risk of heart disease. As little as one serving of oily fish a week may decrease your chance of a fatal heart attack by as much as 40 percent.

Heart disease is a major cause of death in the Western world. While there are many risk factors, evidence suggests that diet can play an important role in protecting against this condition.

There has been a great deal of controversy over the relationship between diet and coronary heart disease (CHD). Aging and hereditary predisposition are risk factors that cannot be altered, but high blood

healthy heart

cholesterol and blood pressure, lack of exercise, obesity, smoking, and diabetes mellitus are all controllable.

Most health experts agree that dietary and lifestyle changes can help. Certain foods have been found to reduce the risk of CHD, while others increase the risk. Recent studies have shown that as little as one serving of oily fish a week may decrease the risk of fatal CHD by as much as 40 percent. These fatty acids thin the blood, helping to prevent blood clots and reduce cholesterol levels. Soy offers similar benefits. Folic acid, found in dried beans and lentils and green vegetables, helps to reduce levels of the amino acid homocysteine, high levels of which have been linked to CHD and strokes. Fruits and vegetables—wonder foods—provide fiber as well as generous amounts of phytochemicals (see page 8), antioxidants, vitamins C and E, and beta carotene. They support the body's defence system and prevent the furring up of arteries that in time leads to heart disease.

Garlic helps reduce blood pressure and cholesterol levels.

USEFUL FOODS

- ✅ Oily fish, including tuna, salmon, mackerel, sardines, and herrings, may reduce the risk of CHD.
- ✅ Garlic supports the cardiovascular system and may reduce cholesterol levels and blood pressure.
- ✅ Oats, nuts, whole grains, and dried beans and lentils provide insoluble fiber, which can reduce blood cholesterol. Oats can also reduce high blood pressure.
- ✅ Red wine (in moderation; consult your health adviser first), apples, tea, and onions contain quercetin, which has been found to reduce the risk of heart disease and strokes.
- ✅ Seeds, walnuts, wheat germ, and almonds provide omega-6 fatty acids, which lower blood cholesterol.

AVOID

- ❌ Fatty and fried foods, particularly saturated and hydrogenated (trans) fats found in margarine and processed foods, encourage the deposit of fatty plaque in the arteries, leading to high blood cholesterol.
- ❌ Excess salt increases blood pressure, one of the causes of CHD and strokes.
- ❌ Refined sugar not only leads to weight gain if eaten in excess but has been found to raise cholesterol levels and blood pressure.
- ❌ Alcohol in excessive quantities is damaging to the heart. You should also avoid smoking and reduce your caffeine intake.

mediterranean sardines

Providing beneficial omega-3 essential
fatty acids, sardines are excellent fuel
for the heart and are much underrated.
Serve with bread, broiled tomatoes, and
a green salad.

Serves 2

Ingredients

4–6 fresh sardines, depending on size,
  heads removed, gutted, and cleaned
3 tbsp olive oil
zest and juice of ½ lemon
1 garlic clove, crushed
1 tbsp fresh oregano, chopped
1 tbsp fresh chives, snipped
sea salt and pepper

Mix together the olive oil, lemon zest,
garlic, oregano, and chives in a shallow
dish large enough to accommodate
the sardines.

❷
Arrange the sardines in the dish and
turn them in the marinade. Cover and let
stand overnight in the refrigerator.

❸
Preheat the broiler to medium. Season
the sardines with salt and pepper and
broil for about 10 minutes, turning them
halfway through. The exact cooking time
will depend on the size of the sardines:
wait until they are golden and crispy on
the outside. Squeeze the lemon juice
over the fish before serving.

feeling great

37

Fresh produce provides protective antioxidants and phytochemicals that fight harmful free radicals and stimulate the body's defences against a range of cancers.

The World Cancer Research Fund recently reported that a staggering 40 percent of cancers could be prevented by healthy diet and lifestyle.

Numerous studies support the argument that eating the right foods can reduce the risk of cancer, and may also play a role in supporting conventional medical treatment for the disease. Similarly, eating the wrong foods can increase the risk of cancer.

protecting against cancer

Cancers strongly linked with diet are those of the stomach, bowel, breast, cervix, pancreas, liver, and mouth. High intake of both soluble and insoluble fiber (see page 10) safeguards against the development of colon cancer and possibly that of the breast. Whole grains, dried beans and lentils, brown rice, and vegetables are good sources of insoluble fiber. Along with beneficial amounts of vitamins C, E, and beta carotene, fresh produce provides a catalogue of protective antioxidants and phytochemicals that fight harmful free radicals and stimulate the body's defences against a range of cancers, including lung, esophagus, and stomach. The antioxidant selenium, found in whole-grain cereals, eggs, seafood, and seeds, has also been found to play a preventative role, especially against breast cancer.

A diet high in saturated and hydrogenated or trans fats may increase the risk of cancer of the bowel, pancreas, breast, and prostate. Opt instead for unsaturated fats such as olive oil and those rich in omega-3 and omega-6 fatty acids found in oily fish, linseeds, nuts, and seeds.

USEFUL FOODS

- ✓ The powerful antioxidant lycopene, mainly found in tomatoes as well as watermelon and pink grapefruit, reduces the risk of some cancers, particularly that of the prostate. It may also safeguard against cancer of the breast, colon, stomach, and lung.

- ✓ Soybeans, tofu, soy milk, and miso contain isoflavones, believed to reduce the risk of hormone-related cancers such as those of the breast and prostate.

- ✓ Green tea (and black tea to a lesser degree) may protect against cancer of the colon, pancreas, urinary tract, and rectum.

Tomatoes are an excellent source of the powerful antioxidant lycopene.

AVOID

- ✗ Red meat in large quantities may increase your risk of colon cancer. Limit eating red meat to 2–3 times a week.

- ✗ Salt-cured, pickled, smoked, charbroiled, or grilled meats and fish have been linked to certain cancers. Eat only occasionally.

- ✗ Cut down on saturated fat, found in many animal protein foods and fried foods. Opt instead for low-fat alternatives.

- ✗ Excessive alcohol intake is recognized as a cancer-risk, as is smoking.

- ✗ Rancid and overheated oils and fats increase the risk of cancer. Don't store oils for a long time and avoid reusing them.

super stir-fry

Fast and fresh, this stir-fry contains
plentiful amounts of cancer-protective
vegetables and seeds.

Serves 2

Ingredients

½ tbsp peanut or vegetable oil

splash of toasted sesame oil

5 oz/150 g broccoli florets

1 scallion, sliced

3 oz/75 g bok choy, sliced

3 oz/75 g fine green beans, trimmed

1 garlic clove, chopped

½-inch/1-cm piece fresh gingerroot,
    peeled and finely chopped

1 tbsp fresh apple juice

1 tbsp soy sauce

1 tbsp sesame seeds

Heat a skillet or wok and add the peanut
and sesame oils. Add the broccoli,
onion, bok choy, and green beans. Stir-
fry, tossing the vegetables continuously,
for 6 minutes.

Add the garlic and ginger and stir-fry
for an additional minute. Pour in the
apple juice and soy sauce and cook for
1–2 minutes (add a little water if the
stir-fry appears too dry) until the
vegetables are just tender.

❸

Sprinkle the sesame seeds on top
and serve.

If you feel run down, include plenty of B-group vitamins and iron-rich foods in your diet and—if you suspect a cold—minimize dairy foods.

Numerous studies confirm the link between poor diet and an impaired immune system. Weakened immunity depletes the body, leaving it more vulnerable to illness and disease.

A diet based on fruits and vegetables (at least 5 portions a day), whole grains, lean meat, poultry, fish, dairy foods, shellfish, nuts, and dried beans and lentils provides a good balance of immune-boosting nutrients

boost your immune system

that will help the body fight infections and stay healthy. Equally important are regular exercise, plenty of sleep, and a positive attitude to life.

The antioxidant vitamin C, found in beneficial amounts in fruits and vegetables, packs a powerful punch when defending the body against colds, flu, and infections. It also encourages the brain to produce endorphins or "happy hormones" that lift the spirits. Other effective antioxidants—which help to protect against illness by neutralizing harmful substances or free radicals in the body—are beta carotene, zinc, vitamin E, iron, and selenium.

If you feel run down, include plenty of B-group vitamins and iron-rich foods in your diet such as whole grains, lean red meat, eggs, dried beans and lentils, yeast extract, dried apricots, and green leafy vegetables. Quercetin, found in apples and onions, also helps to fight viruses and stop them replicating, while horseradish and watercress are good for opening up congested passages. If you catch a cold, drink plenty of fluids to prevent dehydration and eat light meals based on soups and juices to help the body purify and restore itself.

USEFUL FOODS

- ✅ Eat vitamin C-rich foods such as citrus fruits, berries, strawberries, broccoli, sweet potatoes, carrots, and dark green leafy vegetables.
- ✅ Shiitake mushrooms are renowned in the Far East for improving immunity to illness.
- ✅ Garlic has been shown to enhance the immune system thanks to its antiviral and antibacterial properties.
- ✅ Zinc-rich foods such as seafood, poultry, lean meat, whole grains, and pumpkin seeds are vital to the production of antibodies that maintain the immune system.

Treat yourself to some strawberries to up your intake of vitamin C.

AVOID

- ❌ Dairy foods should be reduced at the first sign of a cold. They are mucus forming, encouraging congestion and blocked sinuses.
- ❌ Drinks containing caffeine inhibit the absorption of valuable nutrients.
- ❌ Antibiotics are no use if you have a common cold—they cannot cure viral infections, and can compromise the health of the gut.
- ❌ Processed foods lack the nutrients necessary for a healthy immune system.

RECIPE

immunity-boosting juice

Help the body fight infections with this powerful combo of fruits and vegetables.

Serves 2

Ingredients

2 large carrots

2 large cooked beets, halved

2 apples, quartered and cored

2 oranges, peeled and quartered

1 cup seedless white grapes

1½-inch/4-cm piece fresh gingerroot

❶

Juice the carrots, beets, apples, oranges, grapes, and ginger. Drink immediately. Alternatively, process in a blender or food processor, strain, and dilute with fresh orange juice if necessary.

IMMUNE SYSTEM TIPS

✚ THE HERB ECHINACEA IS RENOWNED AS AN EXCELLENT IMMUNE SYSTEM-BOOSTER, CUTTING THE DURATION OF THE COMMON COLD AS WELL AS ALLEVIATING ITS SYMPTOMS.

The efficient digestion of food is dependent on water: try to drink 6–8 glasses of mineral or filtered water every day.

A healthy digestive system is vital for general wellbeing. If your system isn't working efficiently, vitamins, minerals, essential fats, proteins, and carbohydrates cannot be absorbed by the body.

To break down food effectively, we need a balance of "friendly" bacteria in the gut as well as digestive enzymes. If these bacteria are out of kilter due to poor diet, stress, antibiotics, illness, food intolerances, or toxin

healthy digestion

overload, conditions such as nausea, flatulence, indigestion, and constipation can occur.

Certain foods can help to keep the digestive system running smoothly. Live bio yogurt contains "friendly" bacteria that help digestion, the condition of the gut, and increase resistance to infection, especially following a course of antibiotics. Sufficient intake of fiber reduces the risk of constipation, hemorrhoids, and diverticulitis, an inflammation of the bowel. A diet rich in fruits, vegetables, dried beans and lentils, and whole grains will ensure that you have an adequate fiber intake. Bran, however, can exacerbate some digestive disorders, since it is not fully digested in the small intestine. Water is vital for the efficient digestion of food, as well as rehydrating the body following illness and preventing constipation. Try to drink 6–8 glasses of mineral or filtered water every day.

If you have recurring digestive problems, a food allergy or intolerance may be the cause. Celiac disease, for example, is an intolerance to gluten found in wheat and cereals. Consult your health adviser if you are concerned, particularly before eliminating foods from your diet.

USEFUL FOODS

- ✓ Live plain bio yogurt improves the condition of the gut and alleviates gastro-intestinal disorders.
- ✓ Apples are said to help cleanse the digestive system.
- ✓ Peppermint, ginger, and camomile tea have a soothing effect on the digestive system and replace lost fluids following diarrhea and vomiting.
- ✓ Certain foods such as asparagus, artichokes, garlic, onions, bananas, tomatoes, wheat, and barley contain a type of fiber that stimulates the growth of beneficial bacteria in the gut.

AVOID

- ✗ Refined carbohydrates, including white bread, pasta, and rice, contain less fiber and nutrients than unrefined, whole-grain varieties.
- ✗ Fatty foods stimulate acid production in the gut, leading to indigestion.
- ✗ Alcohol increases stomach acidity and can aggravate irritable bowel syndrome.
- ✗ Wheat bran can aggravate stomach disorders and inhibit absorption of certain nutrients.
- ✗ Curries and other spicy foods can irritate the gut.

Apples have a detoxifying effect on the digestive system.

banana and strawberry smoothie

Bananas can help to prevent indigestion and ulcers, while live bio yogurt boosts and restores the condition of the gut by introducing beneficial bacteria.

Serves 2

Ingredients

2 ripe bananas, quartered

1²⁄₃ cups strawberries, hulled and halved if large

2¹⁄₄ cups live plain bio yogurt

Place the bananas, strawberries, and yogurt in a blender or food processor. Process until smooth and creamy— dilute with a little milk if too thick. Drink immediately.

DIGESTION TIPS

⊕ GO TO PAGE 64 FOR FURTHER ADVICE ON DEALING WITH CONSTIPATION AND IRRITABLE BOWEL SYNDROME, AND PAGE 70 FOR HELP WITH INDIGESTION AND HEARTBURN.

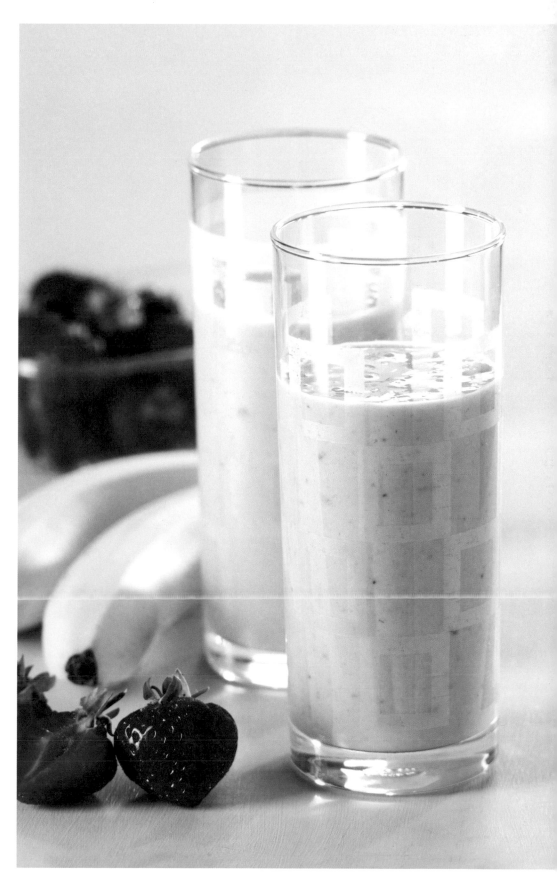

Long-term feelings of anxiety can raise both blood pressure and cholesterol levels, and increase your risk of certain illnesses.

Food has a direct effect on mood. It can induce a feeling of calm or, conversely, make you feel anxious and tense—it's important to get the balance right.

We all suffer from stress at some time or another; it is our ability to cope that varies. Perhaps surprisingly, diet can affect our ability to handle stressful situations, limiting their negative effects on the mind and body.

achieving calm

Not all stress is bad for us, but long-term feelings of anxiety can be damaging, raising blood pressure and cholesterol levels and increasing the risk of certain illnesses and conditions, including irritable bowel, headaches, and palpitations.

The frequency of meals can make a noticeable difference to tension levels. Eating regularly with the occasional healthy snack in between main meals will keep blood sugar levels on an even keel, helping you to avoid mood swings and allowing the body to cope with physical and mental pressures.

Unrefined carbohydrate foods have a calming effect on the brain. They help to transport tryptophan, the amino acid that produces the brain chemical serotonin, a natural uplifter and calmer. The B-group vitamins play a crucial role in how well you cope with stressful situations. They enable the nervous system to function well and help to release energy from the cells, which are under pressure during times of stress. Vitamin C has also been found to reduce levels of stress hormones in the blood. These vitamins cannot be stored in the body for long, so need to be replenished on a daily basis. The minerals magnesium, zinc, and calcium are needed in greater amounts during times of stress and a shortage will affect your ability to cope under pressure.

USEFUL FOODS

- Omega-3 essential fatty acids are thought to have a calming effect during times of pressure. Try to include salmon, herrings, mackerel, pilchards, sardines, or tuna in your diet twice a week.

- Instead of reaching for a chocolate bar, eat some fresh fruit—its natural sugars are released more slowly in the body, providing steady supplies of energy. Fruits also contain immunity-boosting vitamins, essential during stressful periods.

- Replenish stores of B-group vitamins by including whole grains, yeast extract, dairy produce, dried beans, peas and lentils, green vegetables, seafood, lean meat, eggs, and nuts in your diet.

- Foods rich in calcium, particularly dairy products, tofu, seeds, and dark-green leafy vegetables, help to reduce tension.

AVOID

- Stimulants like alcohol and cigarettes rob the body of valuable nutrients, including vitamins A, B, and C, zinc, magnesium, and essential fatty acids. Alcohol is also a chemical depressant.

- Fatty and sugary foods provide few nutrients and also suppress the appetite. Refined sugar in particular leads to yo-yoing energy levels, resulting in more stress and lethargy.

- Caffeine, found in tea, coffee, and soda, inhibits the uptake of iron, calcium, and magnesium. Fruit or herbal teas are a healthy alternative.

fresh tuna niçoise

This twist on the classic French salad provides valuable omega-3 fatty acids, antioxidants, and B-group vitamins, which help to counter stress.

Serves 2

Ingredients

1 tbsp olive oil

1 tbsp fresh lemon juice

2 x 5 oz/150 g fresh tuna steaks

9 oz/250 g new potatoes, halved and cooked

3 oz/75 g fine green beans, cooked

4 oz/115 g mixed salad greens

6 cherry tomatoes, halved

1 small red onion, sliced

handful black olives, pitted

salt and pepper

Dressing

1 tbsp extra virgin olive oil

½ tsp white wine vinegar

1 small garlic clove, crushed

3 tsp reduced-fat mayonnaise

1

Mix together the oil and lemon juice and season well. Place the tuna in a shallow dish and pour over the marinade. Cover and chill for 30 minutes, turning the tuna occasionally.

2

Put the new potatoes, green beans, salad greens, tomatoes, red onion, and olives into a serving bowl.

3

Whisk together the ingredients for the dressing, then pour it over the salad and toss well using your hands.

4

Heat a grill pan or skillet until hot. Place the tuna steaks in the pan, brush with the marinade, and cook for 3–5 minutes, turning once, until cooked on the outside and pink in the center. Brush with the marinade when needed.

5

Arrange the salad on serving plates and top each one with a tuna steak.

STRESS TIPS

✚ HERBAL REMEDIES CAN BE A BENEFICIAL ALTERNATIVE TO PRESCRIBED TRANQUILIZERS. GINSENG HELPS TO COMBAT PHYSICAL AND MENTAL STRESS AND STRENGTHENS THE IMMUNE SYSTEM. ECHINACEA IS A WELL-KNOWN IMMUNE SYSTEM-BOOSTER, WHICH IS DEPLETED DURING TIMES OF STRESS. GOLDEN SEAL IS ALSO HELPFUL.

feeling great

Eat small but regular meals to sustain energy levels and keep your blood sugar levels steady.

Many factors can zap your energy reserves, including illness, lack of sleep, and bad diet. You can improve your energy levels by reviewing what you eat.

Depleted energy can have a detrimental effect, both physically and mentally. One of the best energizers is sleep, which is something most of us lack in varying degrees. Diet is another factor—when feeling stressed and

boost your energy

tired, your digestion slows down and you don't absorb nutrients as efficiently as you should. Eat small but regular meals to sustain energy levels and keep blood sugar levels steady. It's easy to miss meals when you're busy, so opt for healthy snacks such as fruits, brown pita bread with hummus, and vegetable sticks with cubes of cheese, rather than potato chips and chocolate.

Certain nutrients can help boost flagging energy levels. Make sure you get sufficient amounts of B-group vitamins, particularly riboflavin, which converts carbohydrates into energy; vitamin B_6 essential for energy metabolism; and vitamin B_{12}, required for forming red blood cells that carry oxygen throughout the body.

In some cases, fatigue can be caused by a shortage of just one nutrient—iron. Depletion of this mineral reduces the amount of oxygen reaching the tissues. Women with heavy periods are especially vulnerable. Help your body absorb more iron by drinking a glass of orange juice once a day with a meal. Vitamin C also helps to boost energy. Other vital minerals include magnesium, which works with potassium and sodium to ensure the efficient working of muscles, along with zinc, which protects against viral infections that often precede chronic fatigue.

USEFUL FOODS

- Shellfish, particularly oysters, are the richest source of zinc.
- Complex carbohydrate foods, whole-wheat bread, pasta, whole-grain cereals, and brown rice restore depleted energy levels.
- Meat and fish contain beneficial amounts of iron, as do green leafy vegetables, dried apricots, and dried beans, peas, and lentils.
- Useful sources of B-group vitamins include whole grains, chicken, fish, eggs, dairy produce, dried beans and lentils, shellfish, and red meat.

AVOID

- Short-term energy boosters like caffeinated or sugary drinks cause energy levels to soar initially, then plummet. Sugary foods, including cookies, cakes, and chocolate, have a similar effect, leading to irritability and lethargy.
- Alcohol in large quantities is draining on body and mind—although the occasional glass of red wine can revive energy levels.
- Refined carbohydrate foods like white bread, pasta, and rice destabilize energy levels by causing a sharp increase in blood sugar levels.

Increase your energy levels with a seafood supper.

⊕ DON'T UNDERESTIMATE THE POWER OF
EXERCISE: RUNNING, SWIMMING, AND
CYCLING ARE ALL TYPES OF AEROBIC
EXERCISE WHICH INCREASE THE BODY'S
ABILITY TO PROCESS OXYGEN, DELIVERING
IT MORE EFFICIENTLY TO THE BRAIN.

⊕ MEDITATION AND YOGA ARE GREAT
ENERGIZERS AS WELL AS RELAXANTS.
THEY ENCOURAGE US TO LET GO OF
PROBLEMS, REJUVENATE THE BODY
AND MIND, AND PROMOTE A MORE
POSITIVE ATTITUDE.

⊕ RESEARCH SHOWS THAT AN HOUR
OF MASSAGE IS EQUIVALENT TO
3 HOURS' SLEEP—TREAT YOURSELF!

RECIPE

apricot purée

Dried apricots provide beneficial
amounts of iron, beta carotene, and
vitamin C. This purée is very versatile:
add a spoonful to live plain yogurt,
use to fill pies, or serve with cooked
meats. For an energizing breakfast,
stir into porridge.

Serves 2

Ingredients

1 cup dried unsulphured apricots,
coarsely chopped

½-inch/1-cm piece fresh gingerroot,
finely grated (optional)

❶

Place the apricots and ginger in a pan.
Cover with water and bring to a boil.
Reduce the heat and simmer for
10 minutes until soft.

❷

Allow to cool a little, then place
the mixture, including the cooking
liquid, in a blender or food processor
and purée until smooth.

feeling great

Sugary foods are one of the major causes of brain drain, feeding an inconsistent supply of energy to the brain that can actually "cloud" mental activity.

The brain needs nourishment just like any other part of the body. Making positive changes to your diet will not only improve your physical health but also your mental wellbeing.

Diet influences the efficiency of the brain's chemical processes. Even a mild deficiency in just one nutrient can have a detrimental effect on memory, mental energy, and concentration. Pineapples, dried beans and

memory enhancers

lentils, nuts, spinach, and whole-grain cereals contain manganese, which aids poor memory by improving oxygenation and protecting brain tissue, while boron found in broccoli, nuts, apples, pears, grapes, and dried beans and lentils improves mental alertness. Zinc is a crucial brain mineral and is found in shellfish, dark turkey meat, whole grains, beans, eggs, and nuts. Oily fish, including herring, salmon, mackerel, tuna, and sardines, is an excellent brain food, providing omega-3 essential fatty acids vital for the production of brain cells. Omega-6 fatty acids are also essential and are provided by vegetable oils, avocados, nuts, and seeds.

The nutrient choline, also found in fish, is needed together with lecithin to produce the brain chemical acetylcholine, vital for the rapid functioning of memory. The amino acid tyrosine, found in milk, cheese, and seafood, helps to increase mental energy and alertness. Protein foods in general nourish the brain and nervous system, whereas fruits and vegetables provide an abundance of brain nutrients, particularly antioxidants. The B-group vitamins, particularly riboflavin and thiamine, also stimulate brain cell energy and have been found to enhance memory. Eat whole grains, nuts, seeds, meat, poultry, eggs, and green vegetables on a regular basis.

USEFUL FOODS

- Walnuts help to strengthen and nourish the brain since they are a source of both omega-3 and omega-6 essential fatty acids (EFAs) as well as B-group vitamins, iron, selenium, potassium, and zinc. Other nuts and seeds offer similar benefits.
- Fish and shellfish are great brain foods, rich in omega-3, choline, zinc, and B-group vitamins.
- Eggs are a complete protein, which means that they provide all the essential amino acids. They also contain choline, iron, selenium, zinc, and vitamins A, D, and E—a powerful brain combo.

AVOID

- Sugary foods are one of the major causes of brain drain: they cause a temporary surge of blood glucose levels, followed by a slump. This leads to an inconsistent supply of energy to the brain that can actually "cloud" mental activity.
- High-fat foods, especially those containing saturated and hydrogenated (trans) fats, can clog the arteries in the long term, thereby reducing the blood flow to the brain and affecting memory.
- Alcohol and smoking sap energy from the brain by damaging brain cells and inhibiting the absorption of vital minerals.

Eggs provide a range of memory-enhancing nutrients.

RECIPE

honey-glazed salmon

This recipe provides a range of brain-boosting nutrients. Sprinkle with toasted sesame seeds to boost essential fatty acid levels and serve with brown rice and stir-fried broccoli.

Serves 2

Ingredients

2 x 5 oz/150 g salmon fillets, skinned

1 tbsp toasted sesame seeds

Marinade

1 garlic clove, crushed

2 tbsp runny honey

1 tbsp soy sauce

1 tbsp sunflower oil

1 tsp toasted sesame oil

Mix together the ingredients for the marinade. Place the salmon in a shallow dish and pour the marinade over. Turn the fish to ensure it is completely covered. Cover and marinate in the refrigerator for at least 1 hour, turning the fish occasionally.

❷

Preheat the broiler to high. Line the broiler pan with foil and place the salmon on top. Brush the fish with the marinade and broil for about 6 minutes, turning once, until just cooked and still pink in the center.

❸

Place the remaining marinade in a small pan and heat until thickened and reduced.

❹

Spoon the marinade over the salmon before serving and sprinkle with the sesame seeds.

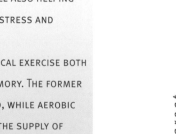

MEMORY TIPS

➕ THE HERBAL SUPPLEMENT <u>GINKGO BILOBA</u> BOOSTS SHORT-TERM MEMORY. <u>GINSENG</u> HAS SIMILAR BENEFITS, IMPROVING ALERTNESS AND CONCENTRATION, WHILE ALSO HELPING TO EASE FEELINGS OF STRESS AND DEPRESSION.

➕ MENTAL AND PHYSICAL EXERCISE BOTH HELP TO IMPROVE MEMORY. THE FORMER STIMULATES THE MIND, WHILE AEROBIC EXERCISE INCREASES THE SUPPLY OF OXYGEN AND NUTRIENTS TO THE BRAIN.

➕ LACK OF SLEEP CAN DEPLETE EFFICIENCY OF THE BRAIN AND MEMORY; TRY TO GET THE HOURS YOU NEED.

feeling great

A nutrient-rich, balanced diet will make for an easier pregnancy as well as ensure good-quality breast milk and a quick postnatal recovery.

Eating a well-balanced diet throughout pregnancy is vital, not only for the mother-to-be but also for the health and development of the baby.

If you are planning to have a baby, good nutrition should be a priority, particularly since a poor diet can make conception difficult. If you are pregnant, now is the time to evaluate your diet and make any changes necessary to give your baby the best start in life. The first few weeks of

pregnancy

pregnancy are crucial in nutritional terms. Don't restrict calories; nurture and nourish yourself and your developing child. Although you don't have to eat for two in terms of quantity, a nutrient-rich, balanced diet will make for an easier pregnancy as well as ensure good-quality breast milk and a quick postnatal recovery.

It is important to boost your intake of folic acid, ideally prior to but definitely in the early months of pregnancy, to avoid neural tube defects in the developing fetus, such as spina bifida. A specially formulated supplement (400mcg) is recommended for the first 12 weeks, and eating the right foods will ensure that you get sufficient amounts throughout the rest of your pregnancy. Iron-deficiency is common in pregnancy, so it is important to eat adequate amounts of lean red meat, dried apricots, eggs, and green leafy vegetables. Zinc and calcium are equally important for the baby's growth. Magnesium-rich foods can prevent muscle cramps, while essential fatty acids found in fish, seeds, and vegetable oil are vital for brain development. Try to eat a variety of fruits and vegetables to ensure sufficient intake of vitamins, minerals, and fiber.

Vitamin C will help your body absorb the iron it needs.

USEFUL FOODS

- Folic acid, especially important pre-conception and in the first three months, is found in citrus fruits, dried beans and lentils, green leafy vegetables, broccoli, dairy products, yeast extract, and fortified cereals.
- Nuts, such as walnuts and almonds, as well as sunflower and pumpkin seeds, provide beneficial oils, zinc, calcium, and magnesium.
- Omega-3 fatty acids, found in salmon, mackerel, herrings, sardines, and tuna, are beneficial to a baby's brain development.
- Calcium-rich foods, including yogurt, milk, green leafy vegetables, tofu, and sardines, will promote your baby's growth.

AVOID

- Alcohol and caffeine prevent the absorption of zinc, low levels of which are linked to nerve abnormalities and low birth weight.
- Unpasteurized, blue, or soft cheeses, soft eggs, or undercooked meat and poultry present a risk of food poisoning, particularly listeriosis and salmonella.
- Foods containing high levels of vitamin A such as cod liver oil, liver, and liver pâté can harm the fetus.
- Peanuts, including peanut oil-based creams, may trigger a reaction to nuts in your baby, especially if there is a history of nut allergy in your family.
- Smoking has been linked to an increased risk of miscarriage.

watercress, orange & walnut salad

Beneficial oils, iron, beta carotene, and vitamins C and E are provided by this simple, refreshing salad.

Serves 2

Ingredients

½ cup shelled walnuts, halved

3 oz/75 g watercress or young spinach, tough stalks removed

1 large orange, peeled and sliced into thin rounds

Dressing

2 tsp lemon juice

½ tsp runny honey

1 tsp Dijon mustard

1½ tbsp extra virgin olive oil

salt and pepper

Lightly toast the walnuts in a dry skillet for 2 minutes until slightly golden. Toss them frequently to prevent burning. Let cool.

To make the dressing, whisk the lemon juice, honey, and mustard together in a bowl. Gradually whisk in the olive oil and season to taste with salt and pepper.

Place the watercress or spinach, orange slices, and walnuts in a salad bowl. Pour the dressing over and toss well with your hands before serving.

HRT offers many benefits, but it is not the only way to get through the menopause, and dietary changes can make a difference.

The menopause affects women in different ways, but for all it is a period of change, both mental and physical. Choosing the right foods can alleviate the range of symptoms associated with this time.

The menopause, when a woman's fertility gradually declines and childbearing years reach an end, usually begins around the age of 50, although it has been suggested that good nutrition and health may delay

menopause

the onset. Symptoms vary from woman to woman: some breeze through with few problems, while others are blighted by hot flushes, insomnia, lack of libido, mood swings, and depression. Hormone replacement therapy (HRT) offers many benefits, but it is not the only way to get through the menopause, and dietary changes can make a difference.

Calcium is vital to keep bones strong and healthy. Bone mass gradually declines during this time due to reduced levels of the hormone estrogen. Vitamins C and D, boron, magnesium, and zinc are also good for bone health. Numerous studies show that phytoestrogens found in various plant foods, such as soybeans, dried beans and lentils, yams, linseeds, and nuts, can relieve many symptoms linked to the menopause, including hot flushes, by mimicking the hormone estrogen. Estrogen has an important role in regulating menstruation and protecting against osteoporosis. Vitamin E also reduces hot flushes.

Weight gain is common during the menopause, but is not inevitable. Stick to low-fat foods, while remembering that seeds, vegetable oils, and oily fish can protect against heart disease and certain cancers, and keep joints and the skin healthy. Zinc, magnesium, B-group vitamins, and tryptophan can help with the common side effects of depression, mood swings, and insomnia.

USEFUL FOODS

- ✓ Soy-based foods such as tofu, soybeans, and soy milk, which are rich in the plant substance phytoestrogens, can significantly reduce hot flushes.
- ✓ Sweet potatoes contain natural progesterone and can help with hormone imbalance.
- ✓ Calcium, in dairy products (stick to low-fat), whole grains, green leafy vegetables, seeds, tofu, seaweed, white flour, and sardines, helps keep bones strong.

AVOID

- ✗ High-fat foods, especially those containing saturated or hydrogenated (trans) fats, increase the risk of heart disease and lead to weight gain.
- ✗ Alcohol, smoking, salty foods, animal protein, raw bran, and saturated fat, and foods containing oxalic acid, such as spinach and rhubarb, inhibit the intake of calcium.
- ✗ Caffeine also inhibits calcium absorption and can increase the intensity and regularity of hot flushes.

Lentils are a good source of low-fat protein, and provide valuable B vitamins.

roasted chinese tofu

Rich in beneficial phytoestrogens, shown to alleviate hot flushes, tofu is best marinated before cooking since it has a neutral flavor. Serve this roasted tofu with stir-fried green vegetables and egg noodles.

Serves 2

Ingredients

8 oz/225 g tofu, cubed

Marinade

2 tbsp dark soy sauce or tamari

1 tsp vegetable oil

1 tsp toasted sesame oil

1 tbsp runny honey

2 garlic cloves crushed

1-inch/2.5-cm piece fresh gingerroot, peeled and sliced

1 red chile, seeded and finely sliced

 Combine all the ingredients for the marinade.

 Place the tofu in a shallow dish and pour the marinade over. Carefully turn the tofu in the marinade, making sure it doesn't break up and that all the pieces are coated. Cover and marinate for at least 1 hour, turning the tofu in the marinade occasionally.

 Preheat the oven to 350°F/180°C. Remove the tofu from the marinade using a slotted spoon and place on a cookie sheet. Bake for 20 minutes, turning occasionally, until golden and crisp on all sides.

 Strain the marinade into a small pan and bring to a boil. Reduce the heat and simmer until reduced and thickened. Spoon it over the tofu before serving.

feeling great

→a–z nutritional healing

The following guide explains how, by eating the right foods and avoiding the wrong ones, you can relieve a selection of the most common ailments and conditions, from acne and arthritis to osteoporosis and PMS. A helpful recipe accompanies the discussion of each condition, along with tips on complementary remedies that have helped other sufferers.

Although there is no evidence that fatty food causes acne, a diet based on processed foods, candy, and snacks deprives the body of essential nutrients necessary for a healthy skin.

acne

Statistics show that 85 percent of people between the ages of 12 and 25 suffer from acne in varying degrees. Dietary and lifestyle changes can play a crucial part in improving this skin condition.

Acne is triggered by hormonal changes at puberty and tends to affect more males than females—although spots are often more prevalent before menstruation. Genetic predisposition may be a factor, but dietary and lifestyle choices certainly contribute. Although there is no evidence that fatty food in itself makes symptoms worse, a diet based on processed foods, candy, and snacks deprives the body of essential nutrients necessary for a healthy skin. Processed foods also tend to include a lot of salt, which has been found to aggravate acne. Try to avoid or cut back on salty foods, as well as seafood, which contain iodine, for 2–3 weeks to see if conditions improve.

A well-balanced, varied diet based on plenty of fresh fruits and vegetables, whole grains, fish, and some polyunsaturated oils is vital fuel for the skin. More specifically, zinc, B-group vitamins, beta carotene, and vitamins C and E are essential. They also assist healing and help to reduce scarring. Including oily fish in the diet will similarly help the healing process and calm any inflammation. Water is vital, since it helps the body to flush out toxins.

Acne may be aggravated by food allergies and intolerances, especially to dairy products. Ask your health adviser for guidance, especially before eliminating foods from your diet. Stress depletes the skin of its natural defenses, triggering a surge in hormones and an increase in the production of sebum, leading to an outbreak of spots. See pages 44–45 for advice on foods that can help to curb stress.

Artichokes and beets have excellent skin-cleansing properties.

USEFUL FOODS

- ✔ Fresh fruits and vegetables are an excellent source of skin-boosting antioxidant vitamins C and E and also beta carotene.
- ✔ Live plain bio yogurt contains beneficial bacteria for a healthy digestive system, essential for blemish-free skin. (Antibiotics, often prescribed for acne, also kill "good" bacteria in the gut.)
- ✔ Foods rich in zinc, such as shellfish, pumpkin seeds, lean meat, nuts, dried beans, lentils, and whole-grain bread, are vital for the skin.

AVOID

- ✘ Milk should be kept to a minimum due its high hormone content.
- ✘ Refined sugar and fatty foods do not cause acne but if eaten in place of healthy, nutrient-rich foods can result in a deficient diet detrimental to the health of the skin.
- ✘ Processed and high-fat foods, which tend to contain high levels of salt, can contribute to acne.
- ✘ Ironically, seafood (see also Useful Foods) contains iodine, which can exacerbate acne.

ACNE TIPS

➕ A DEFICIENCY IN THE DIGESTIVE ENZYMES RESPONSIBLE FOR BREAKING DOWN FATS MAY CAUSE ACNE. THE SUPPLEMENT LIPASE HELPS TO REBUILD DEPLETED LEVELS.

RECIPE

luxury granola

This skin-nourishing granola makes a perfect start to the day served with live plain bio yogurt and topped with sliced strawberries.

Serves 6

Ingredients

$\frac{1}{2}$ cup sunflower seeds

$\frac{1}{4}$ cup pumpkin seeds

$\frac{1}{4}$ cup sesame seeds

$1\frac{1}{3}$ cups porridge oats

$1\frac{1}{4}$ cups barley flakes

$1\frac{1}{4}$ cups wheat flakes

$\frac{2}{3}$ cup raisins

$\frac{3}{4}$ cup roasted whole hazelnuts, chopped

$\frac{2}{3}$ cup almonds, coarsely chopped

$\frac{2}{3}$ cup unsulphured dried apricots, coarsely chopped

$\frac{1}{3}$ cup dried cherries

Lightly toast the sunflower, pumpkin, and sesame seeds in a dry skillet until just golden, tossing them regularly to prevent burning. Let cool.

❷

Mix the toasted seeds with the rest of the ingredients. Store in an airtight container.

Studies show that a lack of vitamin C can contribute to osteoarthritis, but paradoxically, citrus fruits can exacerbate the symptoms.

Early morning stiffness, pain, and swelling of the joints, in varying degrees, are all symptoms of arthritis. Although there is no known cure, certain foods and diet can significantly alleviate the condition.

There are many forms of arthritis, the most prevalent being osteoarthritis, a degenerative condition of the joints that causes stiffness and pain. Studies have found that a lack of antioxidant nutrients,

arthritis

especially vitamin C, is one of the contributing factors. Vitamins A (beta carotene in plants), E, and B_6 are also valuable, as are zinc and copper, for the production of collagen and maintenance of normal cartilage. Paradoxically, although citrus fruits are one of the best sources of vitamin C, they can actually exacerbate symptoms by creating acidity in the body, which it responds to by releasing calcium to create more alkalinity. Strawberries, kiwifruit, mangoes, sweet potatoes, broccoli, and carrots are therefore preferred sources of vitamin C and other antioxidants.

Rheumatoid arthritis is a complex condition thought to be related to a malfunctioning immune system, resulting in severe pain and inflammation that eventually spreads throughout the joints. Recent studies show that the condition can be eased by a largely vegetarian diet based on whole foods, fruits, vegetables, nuts, seeds, and ginger, along with oily fish. An overall reduction in the intake of fat, processed foods, meat, sugar, and refined carbohydrates may also help.

Food allergies and intolerances can aggravate arthritis, although you should consult your health adviser before eliminating foods from the diet. Stress and lack of exercise are other contributors.

USEFUL FOODS

- ✓ Pineapple contains bromelain, a helpful anti-inflammatory.
- ✓ Oily fish and cod liver oil have anti-inflammatory properties and can ease the pain of the condition.
- ✓ Flavonoid-rich berries such as cherries, blueberries, and blackberries can help to relieve symptoms.
- ✓ Foods rich in the mineral boron, including lettuce, alfalfa, peas, cabbage, apples, almonds, and hazelnuts, help the body to absorb calcium and have been found to ease the condition.
- ✓ Turmeric contains curcumin, an effective anti-inflammatory.

Cherries are rich in flavonoids, an antioxidant that can bring relief to arthritis sufferers.

AVOID

- ✗ Members of the nightshade family of foods—eggplants, tomatoes, potatoes, bell peppers, and tobacco—are all known irritants.
- ✗ Dairy products, corn, wheat, sugar, eggs, smoked and preserved foods, coffee, and red meat are known to exacerbate rheumatoid arthritis.
- ✗ Sufferers of gout, a form of arthritis, should avoid alcohol, offal, game, poultry, shellfish, dried beans, and lentils, since they are high in purines, which aggravate the condition.
- ✗ Animal sources of protein contain phosphorus and nitrogen, both of which make symptoms worse.

pineapple & ginger crush

The anti-inflammatory combination of pineapple and ginger in this recipe can help to ease painful symptoms.

Serves 2

Ingredients

1 medium pineapple, peeled and cut into slices

1-inch/2.5-cm piece fresh gingerroot, peeled

crushed ice

Put the pineapple and ginger through a juicer. Pour over crushed ice and serve immediately.

ARTHRITIS TIPS

✚ THE TOXIN-ELIMINATING YUCCA AND DEVIL'S CLAW CAN SUCCESSFULLY RELIEVE SYMPTOMS OF OSTEOARTHRITIS. GREEN-LIPPED MUSSEL EXTRACT, GLUCOSAMINE, AND COMPLEMENTARY THERAPIES LIKE ACUPUNCTURE, MASSAGE, AND OSTEOPATHY, CAN ALSO BRING RELIEF.

a–z nutritional healing

Dark-green leafy vegetables, peas, figs, broccoli, and zucchini provide magnesium, which is believed to protect against asthma by relaxing the muscles of the airways.

Exacerbated by poor air quality and pollution, and allergies to dust, animals, and certain foods, respiratory problems are on the increase. A diet high in fresh fruits and vegetables may help relieve the symptoms.

Like other allergic conditions, including hay fever and eczema, asthma often runs in families. Recent studies, however, show a correlation between wheeziness and a diet lacking in fruits and vegetables.

asthma

People who ate the most fresh produce were also found to have the healthiest lung function.

The beneficial effect of fruits and vegetables is attributed to their high antioxidant content. But fresh produce doesn't only play a preventative role: vitamin C along with other antioxidants, vitamin E, and beta carotene have been shown to ease inflammation of the airways during an attack. Dark-green leafy vegetables, peas, figs, broccoli, and zucchini are especially beneficial because they provide magnesium, which is believed to protect against asthma by relaxing the muscles of the airways.

Vitamin B_6 deficiency is common in asthmatics—avocados, sesame seeds, fish, and poultry may help to reduce the severity of symptoms. Conversely, certain foods may trigger an asthma attack if the sufferer has an allergy or intolerance. These vary depending on the individual—a food that is tolerated by one asthma sufferer may cause an attack in another. A medically controlled allergy elimination diet will help to identify problematic foods. Some asthmatics also react to food additives, preservatives, and colorings.

USEFUL FOODS

- Fresh fruits provide a powerful combination of the antioxidants beta carotene and vitamin C, as well as fiber.
- Green leafy vegetables, like broccoli, peas, and zucchini are a good source of magnesium, fiber, and antioxidant vitamins. Sunflower seeds, nuts, whole grains, fish, and soy also contain magnesium.
- Tomatoes, fresh and cooked, have been found to reduce the risk of asthma.

Tomatoes are rich in lycopene, which promotes healthy lungs.

- Onions, garlic, ginger, and chile can prevent an asthma attack by clearing the airways.
- The B-group vitamins, found in green leafy vegetables, dried beans and lentils, lean meat, eggs, fish, and dairy products, may help asthmatics whose attacks are brought on by stress.

AVOID

- Salt directly affects the muscles of the airways by constricting them. Reduction in salt intake may help to relieve symptoms.
- Preservatives known as "sulphites", added to food such as dried fruits, squashes, wine, beer, hard cider, vinegar, sausages, burgers, jellies,

and some frozen vegetables, can bring on attacks in susceptible people. The food colorings tartrazine, quinoline yellow, and sunset yellow can also be a problem.

❌ Dairy products, wheat, red meat, and yeast may cause or aggravate the symptoms of asthma.

❌ Foods containing histamine, including strong sausages, ripe cheese, and some wines, can trigger attacks in susceptible people.

❌ Saturated fat and hydrogenated (trans) fats may increase the likelihood of asthma.

gazpacho

This classic chilled soup contains an abundance of fresh vegetables, providing beneficial antioxidants.

Serves 2

Ingredients

1 slice day-old bread

1 lb/450 g vine-ripened tomatoes, peeled, seeded, and chopped

1 mini cucumber, peeled, seeded, and chopped

1 small red bell pepper, seeded and chopped

1 green chile, seeded and sliced

1 garlic clove, crushed

1 tbsp extra virgin olive oil

juice of 1 lime

few drops Tabasco sauce

salt and pepper

½ avocado, pitted, seeded, and diced

squeeze of fresh lemon juice

4 ice cubes, to serve

❶

Soak the bread in a little water for 5 minutes. Place the bread with the tomatoes, cucumber, red bell pepper, chile, garlic, oil, lime juice, and Tabasco in a blender or food processor. Add 1 cup of water and blend until combined but still chunky. Season to taste with salt and pepper and chill for 2–3 hours.

❷

Just before serving, toss the avocado in the lemon juice. Ladle the soup into bowls, add the ice cubes, and top with the avocado.

a–z nutritional healing

Antibiotics, stress, the pill, steroids, and a diet high in refined sugars can all cause the candida micro-organism to multiply out of control.

Candida albicans is a yeast micro-organism that lives naturally in our bodies. This normally harmless yeast only causes problems when it multiplies out of control and becomes invasive.

Although candida is not fully understood, it is suggested that nearly one-third of the population in the Western world suffers from candida-related problems, namely

candida

thrush, fatigue, depression, wind, headaches, bloating, allergies, and food intolerances. Antibiotics, stress, the pill, steroids, and a diet high in refined sugars typically cause the micro-organism to multiply out of control. Similarly, problems can occur after an infection or illness, since the immune system is compromised.

When severe, candida flourishes in the gut, damaging, weakening, and destroying "good" bacteria. This is believed to affect the way nutrients are absorbed in the gut and leads to the release of harmful toxins into the body. If the gut and immune system are healthy, the good bacteria in the gut will keep the candida in check. Improving the internal flora of the gut is therefore vital to help curb the overgrowth of candida and subsequent problems. Live plain bio yogurt containing acidophilus cultures eaten on a regular basis is one way to help redress the balance.

Like all yeasts, candida feeds on sugar and starch and sufferers can experience a craving for these foods. Some alternative practitioners believe that people who suffer from recurrent candida-related problems should avoid all foods that contain sugar, yeast, and molds. Ask your health adviser or a dietitian for advice.

USEFUL FOODS

- Live plain bio yogurt contains "good" bacteria that will improve the internal flora of your gut.
- Zinc-rich foods such as whole grains, dried beans and lentils, shellfish, and red meat help to boost the immune system.
- The following foods have anti-fungal properties: onions, cabbage, broccoli, Brussels sprouts, kale, watercress, cauliflower, cinnamon, and extra virgin olive oil.
- Vegetables rich in vitamin C, including broccoli, green leafy vegetables, tomatoes, spinach, and bell peppers, help boost the immune system.

Watercress has anti-fungal and immune-boosting properties that can help keep candida in check.

AVOID

- The following foods have been linked to candida overgrowth: all yeast-based foods such as leavened bread and pizza; alcohol; sugary foods; fruit juices (apart from freshly squeezed) and dried fruits; cheese; mushrooms and fungi of all kinds; pickled and fermented foods, including vinegar, soy sauce, and relishes.

CANDIDA TIPS

- PROBIOTIC SUPPLEMENTS, WIDELY AVAILABLE AT HEALTH FOOD STORES, CONTAIN BENEFICIAL BACTERIA THAT HELP TO IMPROVE THE CONDITION OF THE GUT.

RECIPE

lentil & carrot soup

This nutritious soup makes a filling and wholesome lunch or supper. Serve with soda bread, which does not contain yeast, and a mixed green salad.

Serves 2

Ingredients

1 tbsp olive oil

1 onion, chopped

2 garlic cloves, chopped

1 tsp each ground cumin, ginger, and turmeric

2 carrots, sliced

generous ½ cup red lentils

2½ cups vegetable stock

salt and pepper

2 tbsp live plain bio yogurt, to serve

❶

Heat the olive oil in a pan, add the onion, and fry for 8 minutes until softened. Add the garlic and spices and cook for 1 minute.

❷

Add the carrots and lentils and cook for 2 minutes, stirring continuously.

❸

Pour in the stock and bring to a boil. Reduce the heat and simmer for 40 minutes. Blend or process until smooth and creamy, adding more water if required. Season to taste with salt and pepper and serve with a spoonful of yogurt on top.

Constipation can normally be alleviated naturally: through drinking water, eating correctly, and taking sufficient exercise.

A nutritionally balanced diet can go a long way to relieving most digestive problems, including constipation and irritable bowel syndrome (IBS).

Since the efficiency of our digestive system influences the successful absorption of nutrients from food, as well as affecting our long-term health and wellbeing, it essential to look after our insides. The most common digestive complaint is constipation, yet the problem can normally be

constipation & ibs

alleviated completely naturally: through drinking plenty of water, eating correctly, and taking sufficient exercise. Increasing your insoluble fiber intake is the first step, which is easily done by eating brown rice, whole-grain bread, pasta, dried and fresh fruits, and vegetables. It is best to eat foods that are naturally high in fiber, rather than processed foods that have had fiber artificially added. Each person's fiber requirement varies, so experiment—too much can cause pain and bloating. Increase your intake gradually to prepare your body for the change. Dehydration can also aggravate constipation, so try to drink at least 6–8 glasses of filtered or mineral water a day.

The causes of IBS, characterized by abdominal pain, alternating bouts of constipation and diarrhea, nausea, and fatigue, are largely unknown, but the condition can be aggravated by food intolerance, too much fiber, and stress. Choosing the right foods can help soothe the gut and increase its efficiency.

Boost your fiber intake with nutritious dried apricots.

USEFUL FOODS

- ✓ Unrefined carbohydrates, including whole-grain bread, cereals, brown rice, and pasta, as well as dried beans, peas, and lentils, are a good source of fiber and ease constipation.
- ✓ Fresh and dried fruits and vegetables also contain plentiful amounts of beneficial insoluble fiber.
- ✓ Live plain bio yogurt improves the condition of the gut and promotes good digestion.
- ✓ Peppermint tea and ginger tea may ease IBS.

AVOID

- ✗ Refined carbohydrates, including white bread, pasta, and rice, have a reduced fiber and nutrient content.
- ✗ Caffeine can help to counter constipation in the short term, but it is also a diuretic, which means it makes you urinate more frequently, thereby leading to dehydration. IBS is also aggravated by caffeine.
- ✗ Alcohol and bran can exacerbate the symptoms of IBS.
- ✗ Intolerance to certain foods, particularly wheat and dairy, has been linked to IBS. Consult your health adviser, however, before eliminating foods from your diet.

WORD OF WARNING

⊕ IF YOU HAVE A SENSITIVE GUT OR SUFFER FROM IRRITABLE BOWEL SYNDROME, YOU MAY FIND THAT LIVE YOGURT MAKES THE CONDITION WORSE. CONSULT YOUR HEALTH ADVISER.

RECIPE

exotic fruit salad

This refreshing combination of fruits not only tastes good but is an excellent source of fiber.

Serves 2–4

Ingredients

generous ½ cup raspberries

1 small mango, peeled, pitted, and sliced

1 small pineapple, peeled, cored, and thinly sliced

1 orange, peeled and thinly sliced

½ cup fresh orange juice

1 tsp runny honey (optional)

Purée the raspberries or press through a strainer. Place the purée in a serving bowl with the mango, pineapple, and orange. Pour the orange juice over and stir to combine. Sweeten with honey.

Sweet foods can be eaten occasionally by diabetics but only after an unrefined starch meal or as part of a starchy food.

Dietary considerations are crucial in helping to control diabetes. This increasingly common condition occurs when the body loses its ability to regulate blood sugar levels.

There are two types of diabetes: insulin-dependent and non-insulin dependent. The first signs of diabetes are excessive thirst, frequent urination, weight loss, blurred vision, and dizziness. People who are

diabetes

insulin-dependent do not produce insulin themselves and require regular injections of the hormone, supported by a healthy diet and lifestyle. Those who are non-insulin dependent produce insufficient amounts of insulin or are unable to use what is produced in the body efficiently. This type is most common, particularly in middle-aged people who are overweight. The condition can be controlled by diet and regular exercise, and may also require medication.

If you have been diagnosed with diabetes, your health adviser will guide you on an appropriate diet. Stick to a well-balanced intake of foods (see pages 8–13)—plenty of fruits and vegetables; a moderate amount of whole grains and dried beans and lentils, nuts and seeds, animal protein and essential oils; small amounts of fat; and minimal quantities of sugar. Sweet foods can be eaten occasionally by diabetics but only after an unrefined starch-based meal or as part of a starchy food, as the carbohydrate will keep blood sugar levels steady. Small regular meals, rather than three large meals a day, also help to keep blood sugar on an even keel. Special diabetic foods are unnecessary if you eat a carefully balanced diet.

USEFUL FOODS

- ✅ Whole-grain starchy foods, including cereals, pasta, and brown rice, help to maintain and stabilize blood sugar levels and provide steady amounts of energy. High-fiber foods also reduce harmful cholesterol in the body.
- ✅ Oily fish protect against heart disease, which is common among diabetics.
- ✅ Although fruits contain a type of sugar called fructose, their high fiber content helps to stabilize the release of the sugar into the bloodstream. Vegetables also provide valuable fiber.

AVOID

- ❌ Refined carbohydrates like white bread, rice, and pasta and sugary foods like cakes, cookies, and candy cause sharp rises in blood sugar levels.
- ❌ Saturated fat and fried foods lead to weight gain, a common problem among diabetics. They also increase the risk of heart problems. Opt for low-fat sources of protein.
- ❌ Alcohol in large amounts is a risk. Enjoy in moderation, with a meal.
- ❌ Salt and salty foods increase the risk of high blood pressure, which is common among diabetics.

Refined pasta can lead to a sharp increase in blood sugar. Unrefined pasta helps to maintain and stablilize levels.

RECIPE

The following infusions can help to soothe symptoms of indigestion and heartburn.

mint tea

Place 3 tsp of chopped fresh mint leaves in a cup. Cover with boiling water and let infuse for a few minutes. Serve warm after a meal.

ginger tea

Slice a 1-inch/2.5-cm piece of fresh gingerroot and place in a cup. Cover with boiling water and let infuse for 3 minutes before serving warm. This tea is also good for nausea.

camomile tea

Use a tea bag or place 2 tsp of dried camomile in a cup. Cover with boiling water. Let infuse for 3 minutes before sipping.

INDIGESTION TIPS

✚ STRESS MAY EXACERBATE INDIGESTION, SO RELAXATION TECHNIQUES COULD HELP. LAVENDER, ROSE, MINT, AND GINGER AROMATHERAPY OILS CAN ALL HELP YOU TO RELAX. ADD A FEW DROPS TO THE BATH OR COMBINE WITH A CARRIER OIL AND MASSAGE INTO THE BODY.

a–z nutritional healing

Eating a large meal late in the evening can interfere with sleep patterns. Try to leave 2–3 hours between eating and going to bed.

There is evidence to suggest that what you eat and drink, particularly before bedtime, can determine whether you get a good night's rest.

Up to a third of adults in the US suffer from some form of insomnia, and as many as half say they are dissatisfied with the quality of their sleep. Insomnia is frustrating, exhausting, and can take its toll both emotionally and physically. A good night's sleep makes you feel rejuvenated, more relaxed, and better able to cope.

insomnia

Stress, depression, anxiety, as well as pregnancy and the menopause, can all disrupt sleep patterns, but diet may also play a role. Consider your eating patterns—keeping a food diary will help you discover whether certain meals or dietary habits directly influence your sleep. Eating a large meal late in the evening, for example, can interfere with sleep patterns. The digestive system is not as efficient at night and a large, rich, or spicy meal puts an extra burden on the body. Try to leave 2–3 hours between eating and going to bed.

Conversely, going to bed on an empty stomach may cause you to wake during the night. A meal based on carbohydrate foods, such as pasta, rice, or potatoes, with a small amount of protein in the form of chicken, fish, lean meat, or dried beans, peas, or lentils, is the perfect balance for sleep, while too much protein and sugar may have the opposite effect. Carbohydrates, particularly the unrefined sort, help to maintain blood sugar levels and increase the level of the neurotransmitter serotonin in the brain, which encourages sleep.

USEFUL FOODS

- ✔ A light snack such as a banana, whole-wheat toast, flapjack, or glass of warm milk will keep blood sugar levels steady throughout the night and boost serotonin levels.
- ✔ Unrefined carbohydrates like whole-wheat bread and brown rice and pasta will lead to a better night's sleep than the refined, white alternatives.
- ✔ Herbal teas, particularly camomile, have a soothing, calming influence.
- ✔ Whole grains, seafood, eggs, poultry, nuts, beans, lentils, and dairy foods are a good source of B vitamins, which may influence sleep and play a role in regulating serotonin levels.

Eggs contain tryptophan, which helps in the production of the brain-calming chemical serotonin.

AVOID

- ✘ Coffee, tea, cola, and drinking chocolate all contain the stimulant caffeine, which causes insomnia and dehydration.
- ✘ One or two alcoholic drinks may aid relaxation, but too many can interfere with sleep patterns and cause dehydration.
- ✘ Sugar causes a surge in blood sugar levels that will keep you awake.
- ✘ Spicy and high-fat foods, such as cheese, put a strain on the digestive system, particularly if eaten too close to bedtime.

➕ LAVENDER AND BASIL AROMATHERAPY OILS ARE PERFECT SLEEP INDUCERS. PUT A FEW DROPS IN THE BATH OR ON THE PILLOW BEFORE BEDTIME. HERBAL MEDICINE, INCLUDING PASSIFLORA AND VALERIAN, CAN ALSO HELP.

➕ REGULAR EXERCISE (ALTHOUGH NOT IN THE EVENING) PROMOTES BETTER SLEEP PATTERNS AND AIDS RELAXATION.

RECIPE

speedy tuna pasta

Pasta, particularly whole-wheat, and tuna encourage the production of the sleep-inducing serotonin in the brain.

Serves 2

Ingredients
5 oz/150 g whole-wheat spaghetti
1 tbsp olive oil
1 garlic clove, chopped
½ cup white wine (optional)
1¼ cups strained tomatoes
pinch of sugar (optional)
1 tsp dried oregano
small can tuna in oil, drained
salt and pepper

Cook the pasta according to the package instructions. Drain, reserving a little of the cooking water. Meanwhile, heat the oil in a heavy-bottomed pan. Fry the garlic for 1 minute. Pour in the wine, if using, and boil until reduced and the alcohol has evaporated.

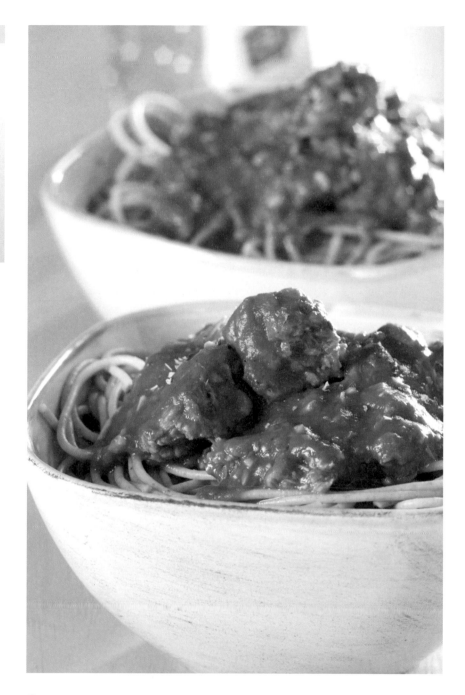

❷

Reduce the heat and add the tomatoes, sugar, and oregano. Cook for an additional 10 minutes. Add the tuna and cooking water and season with salt and pepper. Cook for an additional 5 minutes.

❸

Top the pasta with the sauce and serve.

Both headaches and migraines can occur when blood sugars are out of kilter, swinging from very low to very high and vice versa.

Both headaches and migraines can be debilitating, and the point where a headache becomes a migraine is unclear. What is evident is that diet can have an influence.

Stress, anxiety, dehydration, alcohol, certain foods, and poor eating habits can all contribute to headaches and migraines. Migraines come with a range of symptoms, from severe headache, nausea, and vomiting to

migraines & headaches

blurred and disturbed vision, which may include flashing or zigzag lights before the eyes and a dislike of bright light. They tend to affect more women than men and can be triggered by a number of factors, one of which is diet.

It's a good idea to keep a food diary for a few weeks to determine whether there is a pattern to your migraines. Eating small, regular meals and avoiding certain foods may be sufficient to curb symptoms. Both headaches and migraines can occur when blood sugars are out of kilter, swinging from very low to very high and vice versa. To even out these irregularities, avoid refined sugary foods and, if you fancy something sweet, make sure it contains some fiber so that you experience a steady rise in blood sugar—dried fruits, bananas, oatcakes with jelly, flapjacks, for example. Avoid skipping meals as this will cause a dip in blood sugar.

Foods rich in magnesium as well as oily fish have been found to help prevent migraines and headaches. Food allergies have also been implicated as a trigger: ask your health adviser for a referral to a dietitian to rule out this cause.

Magnesium-rich foods, including nuts, can help prevent a migraine attack.

USEFUL FOODS

- ✓ High-fiber foods, including whole-grain bread, oatcakes, brown rice, fruits and vegetables, and whole-wheat pasta, help to keep blood sugar levels steady.
- ✓ Magnesium-rich foods—nuts, seeds, whole grains, green vegetables, and soy—can help to prevent migraines.
- ✓ Oily fish—sardines, mackerel, salmon, herrings, and tuna—are also believed to help prevent migraines as they have an anti-inflammatory effect.
- ✓ Make sure you drink plenty of water, as dehydration causes headaches.

AVOID

- ✗ Chocolate, hard cheese, sour cream, red wine, smoked and cured fish, and meat contain substances that can trigger a migraine.
- ✗ Caffeine can set off a migraine, so cut down on coffee, tea, and cola—but do it gradually as a dramatic withdrawal can also trigger an attack.
- ✗ Food additives, including artificial sweeteners, nitrates in preserved meat, as well as monosodium glutamate (MSG), used in potato chips, bottled sauces, ready-meals and, by some Chinese restaurants, can trigger migraines and headaches.

RECIPE

mixed herb salad with toasted nuts and seeds

This salad contains beneficial vitamins, minerals, and oils, and makes a perfect light lunch served with crusty whole-wheat bread.

Serves 2

Ingredients

2 oz/50 g mixed salad greens, including watercress and/or spinach

2 oz/50 g mixed herbs, including parsley, arugula, and basil

1 tbsp sunflower seeds

1 tbsp pumpkin seeds

1 tbsp pine nuts

Dressing

2 tbsp extra virgin olive oil

1–2 tsp fresh lemon juice

salt and pepper

❶

Arrange the salad greens and herbs in a serving bowl. Lightly toast the seeds and pine nuts in a dry skillet until just colored. Let cool slightly before sprinkling over the salad.

❷

Mix together the olive oil and lemon juice. Season to taste with salt and pepper and drizzle over the salad.

MIGRAINE TIPS

✚ HEADACHES AND MIGRAINES ARE OFTEN CAUSED BY STRESS. MASSAGE LAVENDER ESSENTIAL OIL INTO YOUR TEMPLES AND TRY RELAXATION TECHNIQUES, MEDITATION, AND YOGA TO RELIEVE TENSION.

Evidence suggests that eating more calcium-rich foods from a young age will help to prevent or slow down the onset of osteoporosis.

What you eat has a huge influence on the condition and strength of your bones. The best approach to maintaining good bone health is a balanced diet combined with regular weight-bearing exercise.

The key years for the formation of a healthy skeleton are between puberty and 30, when bone mass reaches a peak and then begins to level off. With advancing age, the bones of both women and men become

osteoporosis

progressively weaker and prone to fracture. Women are more vulnerable due to their smaller frames and declining levels of the hormone estrogen and subsequent calcium loss during the menopause. Excessive dieting, especially during the key years, has a detrimental effect on the skeleton, since the body is starved of the nutrients required for bone health. Dieting can also interfere with estrogen production in women.

There is growing evidence to suggest that eating more calcium-rich foods from a young age will help to prevent or slow down the onset of osteoporosis. Adequate levels of vitamin D are also essential for the absorption of calcium. Getting outdoors in the sunshine helps the skin to make this nutrient, which is also found in some foods. Magnesium, boron, zinc, manganese, and copper are also needed for good bones. If you eat a well-balanced, varied diet, you should be getting sufficient quantities of all these nutrients.

Regular exercise is just as important for building bone strength, since it ensures nutrients are more readily absorbed where they are needed and encourages new bone formation. Jogging, aerobics, and walking are all recommended.

USEFUL FOODS

- Milk, cheese, and yogurt are good sources of calcium. Opt for nonfat or reduced-fat versions, which contain as much of the mineral as their full-fat counterparts.
- Soybeans, soy milk, and tofu, green leafy vegetables, fortified cereals, sardines, and sesame seeds also provide calcium.
- Food sources of vitamin D include margarine, butter, oily fish, fortified cereals, and eggs.
- Whole grains, nuts, seeds, dried apricots, and green vegetables are a good source of valuable magnesium.

AVOID

- Salt intake should be reduced in those vulnerable to osteoporosis as it increases calcium loss.
- Smoking and alcohol reduce calcium absorption, encourage its loss, and accelerate bone weakness. Smoking also interferes with estrogen production.
- The phosphorus in soda is believed to alter the balance of minerals in the body if drunk in excess, encouraging it to release calcium from the bones.
- A high intake of animal protein can increase calcium loss in the body.

The humble cabbage contains magnesium, which is important for strong bones.

sardines on toast

This simple snack provides plentiful amounts of the nutrients necessary for good health.

Serves 1

Ingredients

2 slices whole-wheat bread

butter or margarine, for spreading

1 can sardines in olive oil

1 tomato, seeded and chopped

sprinkling of dried chili flakes

salt and pepper

1 tbsp chopped fresh parsley, to garnish

Preheat the broiler to high. Toast both slices of bread on one side. Spread lightly with butter or margarine.

Drain the sardines and arrange them on top of the untoasted sides of the bread. Top with the chopped tomato and a few dried chili flakes. Season to taste with salt and pepper. Broil for 3 minutes until golden. Sprinkle with parsley before serving.

OSTEOPOROSIS TIPS

⊕ CALCIUM AND BONE HEALTH SUPPLEMENTS ARE RECOMMENDED FOR MENOPAUSAL AND POST-MENOPAUSAL WOMEN, AND ALSO REGULAR DIETERS.

Certain foods and dietary habits can aggravate or sometimes even cause PMS. Keep a food diary to monitor your moods and physical changes throughout the month.

pms

Making some simple changes to your diet can help alleviate many of the symptoms associated with premenstrual syndrome (PMS).

Premenstrual syndrome is the term used to describe a collection of symptoms, physical and emotional, that occur prior to menstruation and are usually related to changing hormone levels. Symptoms vary depending on the individual but may include irritability, mood swings and forgetfulness, tender breasts, cravings, and cramp—and many more besides. Most commonly, symptoms begin a few days before a period starts and diminish when it begins.

Certain foods and dietary habits can aggravate or sometimes even cause PMS. You may find it useful to keep a food diary to monitor your moods and physical changes throughout the month. The principles of a well-balanced, varied diet apply here. Eat plenty of fruits and vegetables, high-fiber unrefined starches, moderate amounts of protein foods such as fish, eggs, cheese, and meat, and drink at least 6–8 glasses of mineral or filtered water a day.

Deficiencies in vitamin B$_6$ and vitamin E, zinc, and magnesium have been detected in those suffering from PMS, symptoms of which are irritability, fatigue, and mood swings. Mood swings and fatigue can also be caused by erratic blood sugar levels. Try eating a carbohydrate-rich snack during the last two weeks of your cycle. Symptoms of PMS may also be aggravated by food intolerances and candida. If you believe either of these may be a factor, it is important to seek the guidance of your health adviser.

PMS TIPS

➕ SEVERAL SUPPLEMENTS HAVE BEEN SHOWN TO HELP TREAT PMS, INCLUDING EVENING PRIMROSE OIL, VITAMIN B$_6$, MAGNESIUM, AND CALCIUM.

USEFUL FOODS

✓ Vitamin B$_6$, which is sometimes deficient in PMS sufferers, is found in green leafy vegetables, bananas, nuts, poultry, whole grains, and oily fish.

✓ Snacks such as whole-wheat toast, pita bread, cereal bars, flapjacks, or bananas help to keep blood sugar levels steady and prevent mood swings and fatigue.

✓ Foods rich in vitamin E such as avocados, eggs, wheat germ, and cold-pressed oils may help to reduce breast tenderness.

✓ Magnesium-rich foods, including whole grains, shellfish, nuts, and dried fruits, are important inclusions in the diet of the PMS sufferer.

The vitamin E in avocados can help to relieve breast tenderness.

AVOID

✗ Caffeine inhibits the absorption of certain nutrients and can contribute to anxiety and mood swings.

✗ Sugar and processed foods like cakes, cookies, chocolate, soda, and some desserts lack nutrients, destabilize blood sugar levels, and may cause water retention.

✗ Salt and salty foods contribute to PMS and cause water retention.

✗ Alcohol and smoking will only aggravate the symptoms.

✗ Cut down on fats, particularly saturated and hydrogenated (trans) fats found in processed foods.

chicken, avocado & arugula wrap

This nutritious snack can be turned into a main meal if served with a salad and new potatoes.

Serves 1

Ingredients

1 small avocado

1 small garlic clove, crushed

squeeze of fresh lemon juice

1 tsp reduced-fat mayonnaise

1 tortilla wrap

1 small cooked, preferably roasted, chicken breast, sliced on the diagonal

handful of wild arugula leaves

salt and pepper

❶

Coarsely mash the avocado with the garlic, lemon juice, and mayonnaise. Gently warm the tortilla and spread with the avocado mixture.

❷

Arrange the chicken and arugula leaves on top. Season and roll up before serving.

→healing foods directory

Use the Directory to identify the foods that are best suited to your particular needs, to find out the nutrients they contain, how they can help and heal, and when they should be avoided. This information will arm you with the means to make positive changes to your diet.

FOOD	NUTRIENTS	HELPS & HEALS	TIPS
Apple	➲ Vitamin C ➲ Potassium ➲ Fiber	⊕ Removes impurities in the liver ⊕ Aids digestion and encourages natural beneficial bacteria to thrive in the digestive tract ⊕ Good for skin, rheumatism, circulation, and arthritis if eaten regularly ⊕ Effective detoxifier and pick-me-up	❶ Look for firm, unbruised fruits. Try to buy locally grown, in season
Alfalfa	➲ Vitamins A & D ➲ Complete protein ➲ Calcium & phosphorus ➲ Iron ➲ Potassium	⊕ One of the most nutritionally rich foods, valued for its ability to cleanse and rejuvenate the system ⊕ Anti-inflammatory and aids digestion ⊕ Boosts the immune system and relieves arthritis, rheumatism, and bloating	❶ Avoid if you suffer from rheumatoid arthritis ❶ Avoid buying mushy, old sprouts. Best eaten raw. Why not try sprouting your own?
Apricot	➲ Beta carotene ➲ Vitamin C ➲ Iron (particularly when dried) ➲ Magnesium ➲ Potassium & boron	⊕ Good for infections of the respiratory system ⊕ Antioxidant qualities may help to reduce risk of heart disease and certain cancers ⊕ Laxative ⊕ Helps prevent high blood pressure and fight fatigue ⊕ May help to prevent osteoporosis	❶ Look for dried apricots that have not been preserved in sulphur dioxide, which can trigger asthma attacks in susceptible people
Artichoke	➲ Folate ➲ Vitamin C ➲ Potassium	⊕ Aids the digestion process; diuretic ⊕ Protects and regenerates the liver, particularly the leaf ⊕ Reduces cholesterol levels, protecting against heart disease ⊕ Purifying and detoxifying	❶ Look for artichokes with tightly packed, firm leaves with the stalk intact
Asparagus	➲ Folate ➲ Fiber ➲ Vitamin C ➲ Vitamin E	⊕ Diuretic and mildly laxative ⊕ Good for the kidneys, liver, skin, and bones ⊕ Contains the antioxidant glutathione, said to prevent the formation of cataracts	❶ Avoid if suffering from gout ❶ Look for tender, young stems with firm stalks. Eat within 2–3 days of purchase

FOOD	NUTRIENTS	HELPS & HEALS	TIPS
Avocado	◆ IRON ◆ GOOD SOURCE OF MONOUNSATURATED FATS ◆ VITAMINS C & E ◆ BETA CAROTENE ◆ POTASSIUM & MANGANESE	⊕ Improves condition of skin and hair ⊕ Soothes digestive tract ⊕ Good for anemia ⊕ Beneficial fats help to reduce blood cholesterol ⊕ Helps stress and depression	❶ Look for almost ripe fruits and store at room temperature until softened. Store ripe fruits in the refrigerator ❶ Brush with lemon juice when cut to prevent discoloration
Banana	◆ POTASSIUM ◆ FIBER ◆ ZINC ◆ IRON ◆ FOLATE ◆ VITAMIN B$_6$	⊕ Rich in the amino acid tryptophan, known to lift the spirits and aid sleep ⊕ Aids functioning of cells, nerves, and muscles ⊕ Eases high blood pressure ⊕ Soothes the stomach and digestive system, relieving both constipation and diarrhea ⊕ Boosts energy levels ⊕ Helps the body eliminate toxins	❶ Eat ripe fruits; green bananas are difficult to digest and cause intestinal wind
Basil	◆ TRACE CALCIUM, MAGNESIUM, AND MANGANESE	⊕ Aids digestion and helps relieve colic and wind ⊕ Rub basil leaves on insect bites to soothe irritation and prevent infection ⊕ Believed to help clear the mind ⊕ Stimulates appetite and counteracts nausea	❶ Add some fresh leaves to your bath for an uplift
Beets	◆ VITAMINS A, B & C ◆ CALCIUM ◆ IRON ◆ POTASSIUM & MAGNESIUM ◆ FOLATE	⊕ General tonic; supports the immune system ⊕ Detoxifies the liver, gallbladder, and kidneys ⊕ Maintains normal blood pressure and combats anemia	❶ Particularly beneficial when freshly boiled
Black Currant	◆ VITAMIN C ◆ VITAMIN E ◆ BETA CAROTENE ◆ FIBER	⊕ Contains pigments called anthocyanins, which are anti-inflammatory and antibacterial ⊕ Soothes sore throats ⊕ Eases stomach upsets ⊕ Antioxidant qualities help to protect against heart disease, strokes, and certain cancers	❶ Look for firm, glossy berries. Ripe black currants do not keep well, so eat soon after purchase

FOOD	NUTRIENTS	HELPS & HEALS	TIPS
Blueberry	◑ B VITAMINS ◑ FIBER ◑ VITAMIN C	⊕ (Memory enhancer) ⊕ Helps combat cystitis and other urinary tract infections ⊕ Detoxifier and antioxidant with anti-infection and anti-inflammatory properties ⊕ Benefits eyesight; may improve night and light vision; prevent cataracts ⊕ Improves circulation, helping to prevent broken and varicose veins	❶ Like other berries, blueberries may trigger allergies
Broccoli	◑ VITAMINS C, E, B5 ◑ BETA CAROTENE ◑ FOLATE ◑ IRON & ZINC ◑ POTASSIUM ◑ CALCIUM	⊕ Protects against cancer of the lung, colon, and breast ⊕ Inhibits the spread of certain cancers ⊕ High in antioxidants, so helps to reduce the risk of heart disease and strokes ⊕ Antibacterial and antiviral	❶ Lightly steam or add raw to salads to retain the valuable nutrients of this super-veg
Cabbage	◑ VITAMINS C & E ◑ FIBER ◑ BETA CAROTENE ◑ FOLATE ◑ POTASSIUM ◑ IRON ◑ MAGNESIUM	⊕ Raw cabbage juice hastens the healing of stomach and duodenal ulcers ⊕ Anti-carcinogenic cocktail—reduces the risk of stomach, lung, skin, breast, womb, and colon cancer ⊕ High antioxidant levels reduce the risk of heart disease and strokes ⊕ Prevents anemia and protects against stress and infection ⊕ Detoxifies the stomach	❶ Apply dark-green leafy varieties (savoy) externally to soothe leg ulcers, wounds, and mastitis
Carrot	◑ BETA CAROTENE ◑ VITAMINS C & B ◑ FIBER ◑ CALCIUM ◑ IRON ◑ POTASSIUM	⊕ Helps prevent and treat cancer of the lung, prostate, bladder, cervix, colon, and esophagus ⊕ Excellent detoxifier, cleansing and nourishing every system of the body ⊕ Promotes healthy vision, skin, and bones ⊕ Aids the respiratory and digestive system ⊕ Helps ward off colds ⊕ Reduces the risk of heart disease and strokes due to its antioxidant qualities	❶ Surprisingly, carrots are more nutritious when lightly cooked than raw as their vitamins and minerals are more readily assimilated
Chile	◑ VITAMIN C ◑ BETA CAROTENE ◑ VITAMIN E ◑ FOLATE	⊕ Stimulates circulation and helps prevent blood clots ⊕ Eases coughs and colds, clearing congestion ⊕ May protect the stomach against alcohol and acidic food ⊕ Anticoagulant—helps to reduce blood pressure and cholesterol levels ⊕ Stimulates the release of endorphins, the body's "feel-good" chemicals	❶ May irritate the stomach if eaten in excess

FOOD	NUTRIENTS	HELPS & HEALS	TIPS
Cranberry	➲ Vitamin C ➲ Beta carotene ➲ Potassium ➲ Iron	⊕ Helps prevent and treat urinary tract infections, particularly cystitis ⊕ Antifungal, antibacterial, and antiviral ⊕ May help people with kidney stones	❶ Store-bought cranberry juice can be high in sugar, making it unsuitable for diabetics
Dates	➲ Vitamin C ➲ Potassium ➲ Fiber ➲ Iron	⊕ Gentle laxative ⊕ Energizing and nourishing fruit, useful for convalescents	❶ The natural sugar content of dates is preferable to refined white sugar but can still cause tooth decay ❶ Tyramine content may trigger migraines
Egg	➲ Iron ➲ B vitamins ➲ Vitamins A & E ➲ Selenium ➲ Zinc ➲ Good source of protein	⊕ Antioxidant qualities may help to protect against some forms of cancer ⊕ One of the few sources of vitamin B12—essential for the nervous system—for vegetarians	❶ Children, pregnant women, the sick, and elderly should avoid raw or under-cooked eggs ❶ Although eggs are high in cholesterol, a diet high in saturated fat plays a bigger role in raising cholesterol levels in the body
Flax Seed	➲ Omega-3 fatty acids ➲ Vitamin E ➲ Iron ➲ Calcium ➲ Potassium ➲ Magnesium	⊕ Also known as linseed, flax seed is one of the best vegetarian sources of omega-3 fatty acids. Protects against heart disease and some forms of cancer, particularly breast ⊕ Relieves constipation and soothes digestion ⊕ Eases menopausal symptoms	❶ Sprinkle golden linseeds over salads and breakfast cereals
Garlic	➲ Sulphur ➲ Iodine	⊕ Wonder food with anti-cancer, antiviral, antibacterial, and antifungal qualities ⊕ Protects the heart by helping to reduce blood cholesterol levels and blood pressure; prevents blood clots by thinning the blood ⊕ Good for sinus and chest infections, colds, and flu ⊕ Can help diabetics by reducing blood sugar levels	❶ Studies show that eating 2–3 cloves of garlic a day halves the risk of a subsequent heart attack in previous heart patients

FOOD	NUTRIENTS	HELPS & HEALS	TIPS
Ginger	➔ POTASSIUM ➔ CALCIUM ➔ IRON ➔ MAGNESIUM	✚ Aids digestion and is an effective remedy for nausea ✚ Effective against colds, flu, and chest congestion ✚ Reduces the risk of blood clots ✚ Stimulates circulation and cleanses the system	❶ Steep slices of fresh ginger in hot water and sip to fight a cold or soothe sickness
Grapes	➔ VITAMIN C ➔ IRON (PARTICULARLY IN BLACK GRAPES) ➔ POTASSIUM ➔ FIBER	✚ Powerful antioxidant flavonoids help protect against heart disease and certain cancers ✚ Powerful detoxifier, so improves the condition of the skin ✚ Treats gout as well as liver and kidney disorders ✚ Nourishing and strengthening qualities make grapes useful for convalescents as well as those with fatigue and anemia	❶ Wash grapes thoroughly as they are routinely sprayed with pesticides—or buy organic ❶ May trigger migraines
Green Tea	➔ QUERCETIN (AN ANTIOXIDANT)	✚ The polyphenols in green tea help to protect against heart disease by reducing cholesterol levels, blood pressure, and risk of blood clots ✚ May protect against some forms of cancer, including stomach ✚ Antiviral qualities protect against flu	❶ Black tea has similar therapeutic properties but to a slightly lesser degree
Honey	➔ POTASSIUM ➔ MAGNESIUM ➔ PHOSPHORUS	✚ Wound-healing properties if used externally ✚ Antiseptic and antibacterial: soothes digestive problems and sore throats ✚ Cold-pressed honey may protect against hay fever	❶ Do not give to babies under 1 year ❶ Raw, cold-pressed honey has the best healing properties
Lentils	➔ B VITAMINS ➔ FIBER ➔ IRON ➔ ZINC ➔ POTASSIUM	✚ Reduces blood cholesterol levels and regulates high blood pressure, protecting against heart disease ✚ Aids functioning of bowels and colon ✚ Fiber helps to control blood sugar levels ✚ Fights fatigue, anemia, and poor memory	❶ Lentils are high in purines and should therefore be avoided by people with gout

FOOD	NUTRIENTS	HELPS & HEALS	TIPS
Nuts	➔ VITAMINS B & E ➔ MAGNESIUM & MANGANESE ➔ ZINC ➔ IRON ➔ SELENIUM	➕ Essential fatty acids (found especially in walnuts, almonds, and hazelnuts) may protect against heart disease and reduce the risk of strokes. Also vital for tissue development and growth ➕ Vitamin E content reduces the risk of certain cancers	❶ Nuts contain high amounts of fat, although it is largely monounsaturated. Eat in moderation
Oats	➔ VITAMINS B & E ➔ IRON ➔ CALCIUM ➔ MAGNESIUM ➔ FIBER	➕ Effectively reduces blood cholesterol, increasing beneficial HDL cholesterol levels ➕ Eases constipation ➕ May calm the nerves ➕ Helps stabilize blood sugar levels, so useful for diabetics	❶ Porridge oats for breakfast make an excellent start to the day
Oily Fish	➔ OMEGA-3 ESSENTIAL FATTY ACIDS ➔ VITAMINS E & D ➔ ZINC ➔ CALCIUM ➔ IRON ➔ IODINE	➕ Essential for healthy cell function ➕ May protect against some cancers ➕ Reduces blood cholesterol levels, blood pressure, and likelihood of blood clots, lowering the risk of heart disease and strokes ➕ Helps rheumatoid arthritis due to anti-inflammatory properties ➕ Improves circulation and skin disorders such as psoriasis and dermatitis	❶ Eat fresh tuna, mackerel, salmon, herrings, anchovies, and sardines twice a week
Olive Oil	➔ VITAMIN E ➔ MONOUNSATURATED FAT	➕ Antioxidant properties help to protect against heart disease, effectively reducing blood cholesterol levels ➕ Reduces the risk of certain cancers ➕ Eases arthritis ➕ May help liver and gallbladder problems ➕ Improves digestion	❶ Buy the best quality olive oil you can afford
Onion	➔ QUERCETIN (ANTIOXIDANT) ➔ VITAMINS A & C ➔ MANGANESE ➔ IRON ➔ PHOSPHORUS	➕ Reduces the risk of heart disease and strokes, thinning the blood and reducing harmful cholesterol levels ➕ Protects against some cancers, particularly stomach ➕ Antibacterial and antiviral, helping to fight colds, relieve bronchial congestion, asthma, and hay fever ➕ Effective against arthritis, gout, and rheumatism	❶ Healing properties are more prevalent when raw

FOOD	NUTRIENTS	HELPS & HEALS	TIPS
Orange	➔ VITAMIN C ➔ BETA CAROTENE ➔ BIOFLAVONOIDS	✚ High vitamin C content helps to protect against many forms of cancer, particularly stomach and esophagus ✚ Protects against heart attacks and strokes, reducing blood cholesterol levels ✚ Boosts immune system and fights colds and flu	❶ Best eaten soon after peeling, since oranges lose their vitamin C content as soon as they are cut
Parsley	➔ IRON ➔ VITAMINS A & C ➔ CALCIUM ➔ MANGANESE ➔ POTASSIUM	✚ Diuretic and blood purifier ✚ Helps eliminate uric acid, benefiting sufferers of gout and rheumatism ✚ Counters anemia	❶ A useful source of calcium for people who don't eat dairy products
Pea	➔ VITAMIN C ➔ THIAMINE (B1) ➔ FIBER ➔ FOLATE ➔ PHOSPHORUS & IRON	✚ Helps to reduce blood cholesterol levels, reducing the risk of heart disease ✚ Fiber helps to steady blood sugar levels	❶ Fresh peas have to be extremely fresh to be as nutritious as frozen
Pepper (bell)	➔ VITAMINS C & E ➔ BETA CAROTENE ➔ IRON ➔ POTASSIUM ➔ BIOFLAVONOIDS	✚ High antioxidant properties, known to reduce the risk of heart disease, strokes, cataracts, and some forms of cancer ✚ Good for skin and bones	❶ Best avoided by those with joint problems as bell peppers are members of the deadly nightshade family ❶ Red and orange contain more vitamin C than green
Pineapple	➔ VITAMINS A, C & E ➔ POTASSIUM ➔ CALCIUM ➔ PHOSPHORUS	✚ Contains the enzyme bromelain which has anti-inflammatory and antibacterial properties ✚ Relieves arthritis ✚ Aids digestion and improves circulation ✚ May help angina	❶ Fresh pineapple is better for you than canned

FOOD	NUTRIENTS	HELPS & HEALS	TIPS

Pulses (dried beans, peas, lentils)

	NUTRIENTS	HELPS & HEALS	TIPS
	➜ B VITAMINS ➜ IRON ➜ FOLATE ➜ POTASSIUM ➜ FIBER	➕ Lowers blood cholesterol levels by about 20 percent if eaten regularly, reducing the risk of heart disease and strokes ➕ Helps to control blood sugar levels, so valuable for diabetics ➕ Reduces blood pressure ➕ Helps anemia	❶ Excellent source of low-fat protein for vegetarians

Rice (brown)

	NUTRIENTS	HELPS & HEALS	TIPS
	➜ B VITAMINS ➜ IRON ➜ FIBER ➜ POTASSIUM ➜ MAGNESIUM	➕ Helps to control blood sugar levels, making it useful for diabetics ➕ May help with psoriasis ➕ Aids digestive disorders and calms the nervous system ➕ Reduces the risk of bowel and colon cancer and also kidney stones	❶ Brown rice contains more nutrients than refined white

Seaweed

	NUTRIENTS	HELPS & HEALS	TIPS
	➜ VITAMIN B12 ➜ IODINE ➜ CALCIUM ➜ IRON ➜ MAGNESIUM ➜ ZINC	➕ Improves condition of hair ➕ Benefits the nervous system, helping to reduce stress ➕ Boosts immune system and aids metabolism ➕ Iodine helps thyroid function and prevents goiter ➕ Helps to strengthen bones	❶ Dried seaweed is now available in many supermarkets

Seeds

	NUTRIENTS	HELPS & HEALS	TIPS
	➜ VITAMIN E ➜ OMEGA-6 FATTY ACIDS ➜ IRON ➜ ZINC ➜ FIBER	➕ Vitamin E (especially high in sunflower seeds) protects cells from oxidation and improves circulation and normal blood clotting ➕ Reduces risk of heart disease and strokes by lowering blood cholesterol levels ➕ Pumpkin seeds promote good prostate health ➕ Reduces risk of some cancers ➕ Supports the immune system and has restorative qualities	❶ Try to eat a variety of seeds, including sunflower, pumpkin, sesame, and linseeds

Shellfish

	NUTRIENTS	HELPS & HEALS	TIPS
	➜ VITAMIN B12 ➜ SELENIUM ➜ IODINE & ZINC ➜ CALCIUM ➜ IRON ➜ OMEGA-3 FATTY ACIDS	➕ Maintains the nervous system and regulates metabolism ➕ Helps to reduce the risk of some cancers and protects against heart disease and circulation problems ➕ Strengthens the immune system ➕ Known as an aphrodisiac ➕ Anti-inflammatory benefits	❶ Recent research dismisses any link between shellfish and high cholesterol. It may, in fact, reduce cholesterol levels

FOOD	NUTRIENTS	HELPS & HEALS	TIPS
Soybean	➲ COMPLETE PROTEIN ➲ B VITAMINS ➲ IRON ➲ FOLATE & CALCIUM ➲ POTASSIUM ➲ FIBER	⊕ Contains phytoestrogens, known to protect against cancer of the breast, prostate, and colon. Helps to balance hormone levels ⊕ Reduces the risk of osteoporosis ⊕ Reduces blood cholesterol levels and blood pressure ⊕ Eases constipation and helps fight bowel disease ⊕ Regulates blood sugar levels	❶ Tofu, tempeh, and miso are all soybean products
Spinach	➲ BETA CAROTENE ➲ VITAMIN C ➲ IRON ➲ CALCIUM & FOLATE ➲ POTASSIUM ➲ FIBER	⊕ Green leafy vegetables help to reduce the risk of cancer of the lung, stomach, prostate, bladder, and skin ⊕ Rich in antioxidants, reducing the risk of heart disease, cataracts, and strokes ⊕ Helps to regulate high blood pressure ⊕ Fights fatigue and mental strain	❶ Eating spinach with a vitamin C-rich food will help your body absorb its iron content
Sweet Potato	➲ BETA CAROTENE ➲ VITAMINS C & E ➲ POTASSIUM ➲ FIBER ➲ IRON	⊕ Good for the heart ⊕ Reduces the risk of some cancers ⊕ Improves condition of the skin ⊕ Helps to regulate high blood pressure ⊕ Cleanses and detoxifies the system, boosting circulation ⊕ Beneficial levels of iron help combat anemia	❶ The orange-fleshed sweet potato has a higher nutritional content than the cream-fleshed variety
Tomato	➲ VITAMINS C & E ➲ BETA CAROTENE ➲ MAGNESIUM ➲ POTASSIUM ➲ CALCIUM	⊕ Contains the bioflavonoid lycopene, said to prevent some forms of cancer, particularly prostate ⊕ Antioxidant properties reduce the risk of heart disease, strokes, and cataracts	❶ Cooking enhances some of the health-giving qualities of tomatoes, particularly the effectiveness of lycopene ❶ Can trigger migraine, eczema, and mouth ulcers
Watercress	➲ BETA CAROTENE ➲ VITAMIN C & E ➲ FOLATE ➲ IRON ➲ POTASSIUM	⊕ Part of the cancer-fighting cruciferous family (also includes broccoli, cabbage, Brussels sprouts, and cauliflower). Effective against cancers of the colon, rectum, and bladder ⊕ Rich in antioxidants, helping to protect against heart disease and strokes ⊕ Natural antibiotic, boosting the immune system and helping relieve stomach and respiratory problems ⊕ Improves skin problems, including acne ⊕ Purifies the system and stimulates circulation	❶ At its most nutritious during the summer months

FOOD	NUTRIENTS	HELPS & HEALS	TIPS
Wheat	➔ B VITAMINS & E ➔ IRON ➔ ZINC ➔ FIBER ➔ SELENIUM	✚ Fiber helps protect against colon and bowel cancer, varicose veins, hemorrhoids, and obesity ✚ Phytoestrogens in whole grains may reduce risk of breast cancer and alleviate menopausal symptoms ✚ Eases constipation ✚ Wheat grass is a powerful detoxifier and cleanser	❶ Wheat is an allergen and should be avoided by those with celiac disease
Yogurt	➔ CALCIUM ➔ B VITAMINS ➔ PHOSPHORUS	✚ The "good" bacteria in live yogurt suppresses harmful bacteria in the gut, so aiding digestion and relieving gastrointestinal problems ✚ Restores intestinal flora if consumed after a course of antibiotics ✚ Can protect against thrush ✚ May reduce the risk of colon cancer	❶ Choose live plain bio yogurt

further information

WEBSITES

American Academy of Dermatology
www.aad.org

American Cancer Society
www.cancer.org

American Diabetes Association
www.diabetes.org

American Heart Association
www.americanheart.org

Arthritis Foundation
www.arthritis.org

Asthma and Allergy Foundation of America (AAFA)
www.aafa.org

Crohn's and Colitis Foundation of America
www.ccfa.org

The Food Allergy & Anaphylaxis Foundation
www.foodallergy.org

Food and Nutrition Information Center
www.nal.usda.gov/fnic.org

Men's Health Network
www.menshealthnetwork.org

National Eating Disorders Association
www.nationaleatingdisorders.org

National Institure of Diabetes and Digestive and Kidney Diseases (NIDDK)
www.niddk.nih.gov

National Women's Health Resource Center Inc (NWHRC)
www.healthywomen.org

Nemours Foundation Kid's Health
www.kidshealth.org

US Department of Health and Human Services
www.os.dhhs.gov

ADDRESSES

American Academy of Dermatology
P.O. Box 4014
Schaumburg, IL 60168-4014
Phone: 847-330-0230
Fax: 847-330-0050

American Cancer Society
PO Box 102454
Atlanta, GA 30368-2454
Toll Free: 800-ACS-2345

American Diabetes Association
1701 N Beauregard Street
Alexandria, VA 22311
Toll Free: 800-DIABETES (342-2383)

American Heart Association
7272 Greenville Avenue
Dallas, TX 75231
Toll Free: 800-AHA-USA-1 (242-8721)

Arthritis Foundation
P.O. Box 7669
Atlanta, GA 30357-0669
Toll Free: 800-283-7800

Asthma & Allergy Foundation of America (AAFA)
1233 20th Street NW, Suite 402
Washington, DC 20036
Toll Free: 800-7-ASTHMA
Phone: 202-466-7643
Fax 202-466-8940

Crohn's & Colitis Foundation of America
386 Park Avenue South
New York, NY 10016-8804
Toll Free: 800-932-2423
Fax: 212-779-4098

The Food Allergy & Anaphylaxis Network
10400 Eaton Place, Suite 107
Fairfax, VA 22030
Phone: 800-929-4040

Food and Nutrition Information Center, National Agricultural Library,
Room 105
10301 Baltimore Avenue
Beltsville, MD 20705-2351
Phone: 301-504-5719
Fax: 301-504-6409
TTY: 301-504-6856

Men's Health Network
P.O. Box 75972
Washington, DC 20013
202-543-MHN1 (6461)

National Eating Disorders Association
603 Stewart Street, Suite 803
Seattle, WA 98101
Phone: 206-382-3582

National Institute of Diabetes and Digestive and Kidney Diseases NIDDK, NIH,
Building 31, Room 9A04
31 Center Drive, MSC 2560
Bethesda, MD 20892-2560

National Women's Health Resource Center, Inc. (NWHRC)
120 Albany Street, Suite 820
New Brunswick, NJ 08901
Toll Free: 877-986-9472
Fax: 732-249-4671

Nemours Foundation Kids' Health
12735 W Grand Bay Pkwy.
Jacksonville, FL 32258
Phone: 904-288-5750

The US Department of Health and Human Services
200 Independence Avenue, SW
Washington, DC 20201
Toll Free: 877-696-6775
Phone: 202-619-0257

index

acknowledgments

Picture credits

CORBIS:

p.6 Michael Keller; p.15 Stephen Welstead;
Tom & Dee Ann McCarthy; p.26 Jutta Klee;
p.28 Lou Chardonnay; p.30 Lou Chardonnay;
p.32 David Raymer; p.34 Steve Thornton

Author acknowledgments

I would like to thank Cathy Herbert for her meticulous editing. My gratitude also goes to Jason Hook at Bridgewater Books for commissioning me to write this book. Thanks, too, to the home economist, Richard Green, and photographer, Ian Parsons.